D1606685

ADOLESCENT DEVELOPMENT AND PSYCHOPATHOLOGY

Edited by

James B. McCarthy

University Press of America,® Inc.
Lanham • New York • Oxford

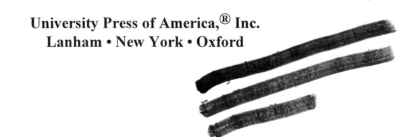

Copyright © 2000 by
University Press of America,® Inc.
4720 Boston Way
Lanham, Maryland 20706

12 Hid's Copse Rd.
Cumnor Hill, Oxford OX2 9JJ

Library of Congress Cataloging-in-Publication Data

Adolescent development and psychopathology / edited by James B. McCarthy.
p.   cm.
Includes index.
1. Adolescent psychopathology. 2. Adolescent psychology. 3. Adolescent
psychotherapy. I. McCarthy. James B.
RJ503.A31436 1999   616.89'00835—dc21   99—051512 CIP

ISBN 0-7618-1565-1 (cloth: alk. ppr.)
ISBN 0-7618-1566-X (pbk: alk. ppr.)

∞™ The paper used in this publication meets the minimum
requirements of American National Standard for Information
Sciences—Permanence of Paper for Printed Library Materials,
ANSI Z39.48—1984

CONTENTS

ACKNOWLEDGMENTS

I ADOLESCENT DEVELOPMENT

II ADOLESCENT PSYCHOPATHOLOGY

III PSYCHOTHERAPY WITH ADOLESCENTS

ACKNOWLEDGMENTS

I would like to express my gratitude to my family, friends and colleagues for their encouragement with this book. I particularly want to thank Ms. Michelle Cruz for her patient work on the manuscript. My thanks and appreciation to each of the authors and publishing companies for their gracious permission to include the following papers.

Anna Freud's "Adolescence" appeared in *The Psychoanalytic Study of the Child*, (1958), Volume 13, pages 255-278, published by International Universities Press. Peter Blos' "Character Formation in Adolescence" also appeared in *The Psychoanalytic Study of the Child*, (1968), Volume 23, pages 245-263, published by International Universities Press. Donald Winnicott's "Adolescence: Struggling Through the Doldrums" appeared in *The Family and Individual Development*, (1965), published by Tavistock Publications, copyright by Routledge. The following four papers were published in *Contemporary Psychoanalysis*: Edwin Kasin's "Youth in Turmoil: An Interpersonal Perspective", (1971), Volume 8, pages 48-60, Donald Meltzer's "Identification and Socialization in Adolescence", (1967), Volume 3, pages 96-103, Murray Bilmes' "Shame and Delinquency", (1967), Volume 3, pages 113-133, and Edgar Levenson, Nathan Stockhamer and Arthur Feiner's "Family Transactions in the Etiology of Dropping Out of College", (1967), Volume 3, pages 134-152. Joseph Barnett's "On the Dynamics of Interpersonal Isolation" appeared in *The Journal of the American Academy of Psychoanalysis*, (1978), Volume 6, pages 59-70, and Owen Lewis' "The Paranoid-Schizoid Position and Pathological Regressions in Early Adolescence" also appeared in *The Journal of the American Academy of Psychoanalysis*, (1987), Volume 15, pages 503-519. August Aichhorn's "Some Aspects of Delinquency: appeared in *Wayward Youth*, (1935), published by Viking Press, copyright by Penguin Putnam Inc. Aaron Esman's "Mid-Adolescence: Foundations for Later Psychopathology" appeared in Stanley Greenspan and George Pollock's (Eds.) *The Course of Life: Psychoanalytic Contributions Toward Understanding Personality* Development, (1980), Volume 2, published by the National Institute of Mental Health Press. Samuel Ritvo's "Late Adolescence: Developmental and Clinical Considerations" appeared in *The Psychoanalytic Study of the Child (1971)*, Volume 15, pages 241-263, published by Yale University Press. James Masterson's "The Borderline Adolescent: An Object Relations View," appeared in *Adolescent Psychiatry*, (1978), Volume 6, pages 344-359, published by the University of Chicago Press. Aaron Esman's "A Developmental Approach to the Psychotherapy of Adolescents" also appeared in *Adolescent Psychiatry*, (1985), Volume 12, pages 119-133, published by the University of Chicago Press. Rudolf Ekstein's "Psychotic Adolescents and Their Quest for Goals" appeared in *The Challenge: Despair and Hope in the Conquest of Inner Space*, (1971), published by

Brunner Mazel for the Reiss Davis Child Study Center.

For Katherine McCarthy and David McCarthy

ADOLESCENT DEVELOPMENT AND PSYCHOPATHOLOGY

CHAPTER ONE
INTRODUCTION
Developmental Theories of Adolescence

James McCarthy

The psychoanalytic theories of adolescence emanated from a developmental psychology that had been radicalized by Freud's heralding of infantile sexuality. Even though Freud wrote relatively little about the personality transformations of adolescence, he elaborated the impact of puberty on both the adolescent's Oedipal complex and character consolidation. In the decades since the 1905 publication of Freud's "*Three Essays on Sexuality*", psychodynamic theories of adolescent psychopathology have been linked to the developmental models of the psychoanalytic orientations. The seminal papers in this collection illustrate the evolution of both metapsychology and clinical theory from a classical Freudian structural model of the mind to the ethos of a developmental and relational or interpersonal perspective. With three exceptions these papers were all written before 1980. They were selected because of their rich contributions to the psychology of adolescence and the analytic treatment of adolescent patients. They offer an overview of the increasing emphasis in theory and practice on the disturbed adolescent's developmental and family processes as well as the subtle interplay of the adolescent's object relations and emotional experience with the analyst.

This introductory chapter examines similarities and differences between Freudian, interpersonal and object relations views of adolescent development and psychopathology that are elucidated in sections I and II. As a prelude to section III of these collected papers, I also discuss aspects of Freud's case of Dora. My discussion emphasizes the analytic exploration of adolescents' primitive annihilation anxieties as a foundation for promoting their healthy character change. My focus on adolescent development and psychopathology does not include a fully comprehensive examination of either psychopathology and cultural or gender issues, or the plethora of adolescent developmental changes. In spite of these limitations, as a way of contrasting the richness of the Freudian, interpersonal and object relations developmental models, I briefly survey essential concepts in the psychologies of adolescence of Freud, Anna Freud, Erikson, Blos, Sullivan, Fromm, Winnicott and other theorists. Although Kohut's followers (Wolf, 1982) characterized the transformation of the self object as the main task of adolescence, I do not summarize self psychology views of adolescence as a distinctly separate theory. Despite their marked differences, psychoanalytic theorists from each orientation have been concerned with the maturational tasks and object relations conflicts underlying the adolescent's individuation process and their expression in character pathology. Contemporary Freudian, object relations and interpersonal clinical theories are congruent to the extent that they underscore the analyst's role in facilitating developmental processes and individuation from internal objects.

Freudian Theories of Adolescent Development

The classical psychoanalytic investigation of adolescence began with Freud's *Three Essays on Sexuality* which affirmed the crucial significance of infantile sexuality for adolescents' establishment of new sexual objects and new sexual aims. Here, as in other writings, Freud stated that the adolescent's character was basically determined by the outcome of the Oedipal period. As a result of puberty, infantile sexuality fell into its final form in such a way that the adolescent's instinctual life became subordinated to the genitals. At puberty, he suggested, increased stimulation of the erotogenic zones coincided with the attainment of genital primacy and an intensification of libido, since the adolescent was capable of finding an appropriate sexual object. Following puberty, a readjustment of defenses was necessary because of the revival of Oedipal fantasies and attachments. Due to their increased instinctual conflicts, adolescents were said to make considerable use of repression, as well as, reaction formation and sublimation. The course of earlier Oedipal development determined the individual's psychological progress throughout adolescence. However, except in cases of what Freud considered to be disturbances of psychosexual development, adolescents' pleasure seeking entailed a detachment from the incestuous Oedipal objects. These changes in adolescents' sexual organization, together with the renewed resolution of the Oedipus complex, conjured up the tasks of character reorganization.

Key adolescent developmental changes in sexual identity and masturbation fantasies were also formulated by Freud. According to his theoretical approach, a reorientation of the body ego and a consolidation of the sexual identity took place during adolescence. As a result of the simultaneous revival and repudiation of Oedipal longings, a detachment from parental authority was likewise said to occur. Although changes in adolescents' object relations were contained in Freud's outline of adolescence, adolescents' object relations patterns were more fully discussed by Anna Freud, Peter Blos and Edith Jacobson. Beginning with Freud's statements, masturbation fantasies were investigated as essential reflections of adolescent development. Freud theorized that, as the agent of infantile sexuality, masturbation took on additional significance following adolescents' intensification of their instinctual drives. Masturbation reorganized adolescents' sexual fantasies in accordance with their erotic attachments and the prospect of genitality. As an outgrowth of Freud's theory, later Freudian theorists, especially Erikson, refocused the theory of psychosexual development to reflect adolescents' ego changes and establishment of a more stable identity. Adolescents' difficulties with giving up Oedipal ties were considered in classical Freudian theory as crucial to the origins of psychopathology. More contemporary Freudian theorists have expanded the exploration of middle and late adolescence, together with these stages' activation of mood shifts and pre-Oedipal conflicts (Esman 1980). Their descriptions of adolescents' failures to relinquish Oedipal bonds have exceeded Freud's focus on puberty as the definitive experience which provided sexuality with its final shape. Ernest Jones (1922) summarized Freud's original view of adolescence with the succinct statement that it represented the recapitulation of Oedipal development. This idea-that infantile sexuality fixed the course of adolescent psychic development - was reiterated in the early psychoanalytic papers on adolescent treatment and character disturbance. Freudian approaches to analytic treatment with adolescents evolved from Freud's view of adolescence as primarily a transitional stage to adult sexuality. Freud's writings only partially emphasized adolescents' emotional lability and their process of disengagement from the family in pursuit of a personal identity.

Anna Freud conducted the first analytic work with children, and she provided the first complete psychoanalytic report of adolescents' emotional instability. Anna Freud's major contributions to the subject of adolescence began with her observations about the curtailment of the truce between the ego and id at the end of the latency period. Her accounts of adolescents' personality reorganization placed great emphasis on regression which stemmed from the need to repudiate Oedipal wishes. She believed that adolescent patients provided analysis with the clearest picture of the dynamic role of both anxiety and the failure of repression in mental breakdown. Her impression that adolescents had only a limited ability to form transferences due to their minimal libidinal investment in the analyst led to questions about the suitability of adolescents for the psychoanalytic experience. In her (1937) seminal work on the ego, she advocated the analysis of defenses before content, and she championed the view that the ego deals with reality conflicts, not just drives. The degree of importance Anna Freud placed on adolescents' regression had the cumulative effect of dominating the classical Freudian conception of adolescent development.	In her classic 1958 paper, *Adolescence,* Anna Freud discussed adolescents' defensive processes as the basis for the consolidation of character traits. By highlighting the defenses, which adolescent patients use in their libidinal conflicts, she continued Freud's concept of symptoms as compromise accommodations with the drives. In particular, she identified three defensive processes as central to the adolescent's character formation. These defensive operations included the displacement of libido, for example in romanticized crushes, reversal of affect or reaction formation, and regression or withdrawal of libido into the self. As a result of the equation Anna Freud made between adolescence and developmental disturbance, the Freudian theory of adolescence illuminated the closeness of adolescents' emotional volatility to the signs of illness.	Adolescents' emotional lability, their susceptibility to anxiety, and their contradictory emotional states were thus all understood as approximations to symptoms.

Anna Freud's description of the incapacities of narcissistic and borderline patients, as problems in early development, was highly influential in increasing the scope of psychoanalytic patient populations. Her (1965, 1980) suggestions about the analysis of adolescents' resistances were based on great sensitivity to adolescents' fears of their regressive tendencies. She believed that if the analyst was able to formulate a treatment alliance, then adolescent patients could be assisted with restoration to the path of normal development. Anna Freud's theoretical writings on adolescence elaborated Freud's view that instincts from childhood developmental phases persisted in the libidinal foundation of character. In her theory the relative success or failure of defenses against Oedipal and pre-Oedipal object ties largely determined the outcome of character. The image she presented of the highly rebellious, regressed adolescent in great mental distress has been challenged by a number of theorists, such as Masterson (1967, 1974, 1978), who have questioned its universality. In general, classical Freudian theorists' accounts of adolescence have stressed the final structuring of the personality in relation to Oedipal and separation conflicts that intensify with the increased complexity of the ego which takes place with the recognition of the approaching tasks of adulthood.

Ego Psychology and Adolescent Development

Enlivened by their association with Anna Freud in Vienna, Erik Erikson, August Aichhorn and Peter Blos all extended Freud's instinctual theory of adolescence, as well as Anna Freud's focus on ego processes during adolescent development. In Erikson's theoretical papers and imaginative biographies he orchestrated a comprehensive psychological approach to adolescent development. By emphasizing the ego's concerns with reality and society, he embellished drive theory, while he created a link to the suppositions of interpersonal theory and object relations theories. Erikson combined psychosexual theory with Anna Freud's ideas about defenses in his well known sequence of the epigenetic stages of human life. In the late 1970's Erikson admitted that the developmental tasks of these detailed epigenetic stages could not be fully realized in any one life stage, since the bases for their accomplishment lay in all of the stages. For Erikson, the psychosexual stages concerned zones for relating to objects, and they entailed unconscious expressions of the child's needs. His psychoanalytic psychology of adolescence was based on the twofold importance of identity formation and the ego's adjustments to the drives and to society. Erikson's writings on adolescence addressed both the anxiety inherent in the process of identity formation, and the analytic task of helping the adolescent to assess values and choices from the point of view of identity synthesis. In contrast to Anna Freud's concern with adolescents' regression, Erikson emphasized adolescents' unfolding maturation and adaptation. In contrast to the interpersonal theorists' belief that cultural forces produced the manifestations of psychopathology, Erikson stressed the influence of societal factors on the ego. Although he retained the tenets of drive theory, Erikson shared the interpersonal theorists' interest in the effect of social forces on psychological adjustment. In terms which reiterated a point that had been made previously by W. Reich, Erikson stated that a society's values had a great impact on the individual's character traits. Neuroses, he felt, or other types of disorders, were expressed in the mental concerns, as well as the physical, and social, attitudes of the person. However, it was the drives that accounted for the enhancement of the child's object relations and the development of his or her ego capacities. The touchstones of Erikson's developmental theory attributed the dynamics of human behavior to the effects of maturational processes, which, he summarized, as man's biopsychosocial unity.

Throughout decades of his work, Erikson crafted a portrait of the emotional, sexual and social aspects of the process of coming of age. In an early (1956) paper on ego synthesis and a later work on the subject of youth, Erikson (1968A) presented a picture of identity growth as stemming from transitory identity crises. During adolescence these passing disturbances were capable of reaching temporary neurotic or psychotic proportions. Identity crises occurred because infantile conflicts had to be reconciled with the complexities of later identifications. Through the concepts of the identity crisis and identity confusion or identity diffusion, Erikson (like Sullivan) attempted to understand the poorly differentiated self and the unsuccessful adaptations of late adolescence. Identity confusion was characterized by difficulties with "intimacy, industry and time perspective". A number of authors, such as Kernberg (1976), have criticized Erikson for not distinguishing the emotional distress of adolescence from the symptoms of serious identity diffusion which earmark the borderline personality disorder. Because of Erikson's reluctance to have young people labelled, as deviant, he argued that adolescents' acute depression, violence, and delinquency all might represent fleeting crises rather than signs of breakdown or character disturbance. Based on Erikson's criteria, follow up studies of adolescents, who exhibited severe identity confusion, have reported its far from transitory nature (Josselson, 1987).

In a highly important paper on identity, Erikson (1968B) contrasted the subjective sense of personal continuity with those aspects of identity which have both individual and social components. His concept of the ego identity referred to both continuity over time and to inner continuity in the face of social patterns and the drives. What Erikson called psychosocial identity was determined by the end of the adolescent period. This latter process of identity formation included the repudiation and assimilation of childhood identifications in a configuration which relied on societal recognition. As a more or less completed process, identity formation thus included the adolescent's most vibrant values and world views which were backed up by societal ideals. Early adulthood signified both a mental maturity and a sexual maturity which coincided with the seeking of new partners and goals.

Erikson's (1959A, 1959B) papers on late adolescence affirmed the active searching for ideals and self images which characterize this developmental stage. The body of Erikson's work pointedly captured adolescents' growing awareness of their personal history and their emergent sense of "I". His theoretical emphasis on adolescents' identity formation has been continued by other Freudian theorists who have connected identity formation with the continuity of self representations (Sandler, 1981) along spatial, temporal and social developmental axes (Grinberg & Grinberg, 1974). However, by making ego enhancement and the establishment of the identity the essential tasks of adolescence, Erikson set his theory apart from those theoretical models which emphasize interpersonal or object relations patterns during adolescence. What Erikson included under the study of identity, other psychoanalytic theorists also discussed as issues of character disturbance and the psychopathology of object relations. Wallerstein (1998) recently noted that although Erikson's work has not been fully integrated into contemporary theories due to his use of structural terminology, Erikson's concept of the ego identity served as an important forerunner of current psychoanalytic emphasis on the self and object relations.

Blos (1962, 1971, 1972, 1980) applied Mahler's theory of separation-individuation, and its concentration on ego development, to the adolescent period. His descriptions of adolescents' object relations and his clinical insights have provided major contributions to Freudian developmental theory. Blos assessed adolescent's changes in object relations in terms of both separation anxiety and the mourning of the preOedipal parents as lost love objects. His (1967, 1968) notion of identity formation was that the more or less completed identity resulted from the integration of self representations into the remainder of the ego. Based on his extensive clinical experience, Blos articulated the goals of analytic treatment for adolescent patients in developmental terms. Successful analytic therapy required the patient's ability to tolerate a degree of anxiety and depression, in addition to the recognition of conflicts and self-deceptions. The most complex, difficult therapeutic goal consisted of assisting the adolescent patient with the deidealization of the self and the deidealization of the object. The mourning of the parents and the reworking of Oedipal conflicts inevitably entered into the treatment process. Blos suggested that adolescents' striving for independence from the internalized objects constituted the second separation-individuation process. Like Anna Freud, Blos maintained that adolescents inevitably regress in order to face their infantile conflicts with internal objects. In accordance with Freud's models of mental life, Blos hypothesized that adolescence draws a line of demarcation between character traits and character synthesis. Like Anna Freud, he saw adolescents' impulsivity and their idealism as evanescent characteristics. According to Blos's clinical approach, analytic treatment with adolescents demanded a lengthy course of therapy. Their difficulty in forming the transference neurosis created impediments to a full analysis of their transference states. Blos (1980) summarized his view of adolescent maturation as consisting of the attainment of ego continuity together with the disengagement from

Oedipal and preOedipal ties. The basic aim of analytic therapy for adolescents consisted of the redirection of the developmental process.

Blos discussed character development during adolescence from two vantage points. In his clinical studies, he consistently listened for evidence suggestive of symptoms in formation as a prelude to character disturbance. In several theoretical papers, he outlined aspects of character formation which were mostly completed by the end of adolescence. Based on the model of Freud, Abraham and Reich, Blos (1967, 1968, 1977) traced the evolution of adolescents' drive fixations into character trends. Character synthesis referred to the structural changes which ended adolescence. The preconditions for this final stage of character formation included the establishment of ego continuity, and the sexual identity, as well as the loosening of preOedipal object ties. Blos conceived of character synthesis as involving the broadening of the ego's autonomy and its ability to handle the aftereffects of trauma. Residual trauma was the chief organizing force in adolescent character formation. Character was therefore synonymous with the pattern of the adolescent's responses and evolving adaptations to signal anxiety. A concise far-reaching summary of Blos's work was contained in his statement that character consisted of the adolescent's ongoing adaptation to residual trauma.

Freud's (1905A, 1905B) clinical descriptions of adolescent patients sketched the charactological changes that follow puberty in the light of his structural theory. The range of structural personality changes during middle and late adolescence has been delineated in detail by Anthony (1976), Esman (1985), Giovacchini (1975) and Ritvo (1971). The conceptual landscape of Freud's psychoanalytic theory of adolescence has also been greatly enriched by M. and E. Laufer's (1968, 1981, 1984) reports of adolescents' body experience as the arena for their developmental and object relations conflicts. The Laufers combined Freud's concentration on puberty and Anna Freud's concept of developmental lines with their own idea that a breakdown in the developmental process, specifically in the sexual identity, was the crucial dimension of adolescent psychopathology. They have consistently noted that the adolescent's distorted relationship with his or her sexual body becomes manifest in pregenital masturbation fantasies that record breakdowns in development. This disturbed relationship with the sexual body represents the primary obstacle to the developmental process. Under these circumstances a poor integration into mature genitality takes place with expressions of shame, and rejection, or even hatred, of the sexual body. For the Laufers, the developmental breakdown constitutes the central aspect of adolescents' psychopathology. This kind of breakdown potentially includes attacks on both the internalized parent and the sexual body. Such expressions of self-hatred have been noted in adolescents' addictions, their eating disorders, and their suicidal self-destructiveness. The Laufers advocate treatment principles based on their exploration of the rigidity of adolescents' defenses, and whether or not the defenses allow for any developmental progress. In their view, the analytic experience facilitates adolescents' detachment from their parents in addition to their resolution of earlier Oedipal conflicts.

The Laufers, Aichhorn, Blos, Erikson and Anna Freud all expanded Freud's vision of infantile sexuality as the cornerstone of adolescents' character formation. While Aichhorn (1935) developed pioneering applications of Freud's theories with young delinquents, Redl and Wineman (1951) and Ekstein (1971) also extended Freud's work to the analytic relationship with severely disturbed, impulse ridden and psychotic adolescents.

Interpersonal Theories of Adolescent Development

Sullivan's (1940, 1953) concepts of anxiety and sexuality placed him at great odds with the Freudian view of adolescent development. His analysis of the pain of his own adolescent years influenced both his theoretical model and his clinical theory of psychotherapy. The loneliness and prejudice Sullivan endured led to his identification of culture and the family as the determinants of psychopathology. As an outgrowth of Sullivan's sensitivity to primitive anxiety, he hypothesized that adolescence was the stage of the greatest closeness to schizophrenia, and he achieved highly effective therapeutic results with adolescent schizophrenic patients. His one-genus postulate enhanced his assumption that the knowledge of psychotic processes was universal, especially during adolescence. His belief that adolescent warps in interpersonal relationships created unhealthy character trends illustrated the neoFreudian belief in the cultural sources of developmental and neurotic conflicts.

The cultural approach to neurotic character formation was shared by Horney and Fromm. Sullivan's view of anxiety, as always being interpersonal in its origin and manifestations, bore a close resemblance to both Horney's (1937, 1939, 1951) concept of basic anxiety and Fromm's concept of existential anxiety as the underlying sources of neurotic character. Fromm (1941, 1947) cautioned that attributing libidinal terms to character traits missed the essential role of the child or adolescent's life experience and family environment. Fromm held that character provided the young person with a distinct identity and a frame of orientation for life. Character evolved through culturally based processes of socialization and assimilation. Unhealthy, destructive character trends, like violence or excessive acquisitiveness, corresponded to both impaired relatedness and the surrender of individuality. According to Fromm, all pathological character traits arose from man's fear of aloneness. The healthy adolescent or adult embraced existential anxiety as a choice over the neurotic, nonproductive types of character orientation (such as the hoarding, exploitative or receptive characters). Sexuality especially registered the extent of the individual's character problems and degree of self-alienation. Singer (1965) extended Fromm's theoretical position, with his belief that sexuality expressed the interpersonal aspects of an individual's pathology.

According to Sullivan, primitive anxiety played its key role in character evolution by creating disabling states of panic and incapacities in interpersonal relations. Like the other interpersonal theorists, Sullivan suggested that neither childhood, nor adolescent trauma indelibly shaped character because life events had a reparative effect on all developmental stages. In keeping with his hopeful outlook, Sullivan concluded that the adolescent stages, particularly preadolescence, proffered the greatest opportunities for the corrections of the deficiencies of prior developmental stages. Within this interpersonal, humanistic model, adolescents' symptoms and signs of character disturbance needed to the appreciated as adaptations to both neurotic values and the cultural processes (Thompson, 1964).

The hopefulness implicit in Sullivan's theory of adolescence was expressed, not only in his developmental outline, but also in his clinical approach to psychotherapy. According to his interpersonal theory, the major developmental tasks of adolescence entailed the attainment of intimacy and the establishment of the lust dynamism. Sullivan (1953) defined lust, the felt aspects of sexuality, as including a pattern of overt and covert symbolic processes. These symbolic processes reflected deep-seated attitudes about oneself and others, rather than infantile sexuality. The negotiation of the tasks of lust and intimacy molded the adolescent's emotional and social adjustment. However, the psychological outcome of adolescence depended greatly upon chance factors, as well as socioeconomic variables, and cultural conditions. The patient's developmental history provided the point of reference for his therapeutic inquiry. The prognostic outcome of therapy could, therefore, be hopeful   even with severe disturbances, because personality never remained fixed, either before or after adolescence. Sullivan alluded to this innate tendency as the tendency towards personality integration.

The centrality of experience for character consolidation during adolescence has been discussed by many interpersonal theorists who have noted the shift away from the dominance of drive theory in psychoanalytic personality theory. Although Barnett's (1978 A,B; 1980) writings did not specifically focus on adolescence, one of his critically important papers is included in Section II of this Volume. According to Sullivan's model, the adolescent stages represented an epoch of intrinsic potential for overcoming loneliness and isolation. Barnett greatly enhanced the interpersonal model of adolescence and character formation with his emphasis on the developmental impact of the dread of interpersonal isolation in character formation and his observation that the self, and its expression in character, was manifest in all of one's transactions with others. In an essay on the importance of shame in delinquency, Bilmes (1967) extended the interpersonal model and anticipated self psychology concepts by connecting delinquent adolescents' shame anxiety and their resulting fear of rejection and isolation with their antisocial actions.

For Sullivan, the attainment of emotional maturity during adolescence was signaled by the degree of healthy involvement in interpersonal experience. The adolescent achieved character consolidation with the increased complexity of his or her organization of experience. For contemporary interpersonal theorists, such as Kasin (1971), Levenson, Stockhamer and Feiner (1967), familial and societal disturbances have influenced adolescents' psychopathology by giving rise to their denial of healthy neediness and their dissociation of authentic self experience.

Object Relations Theories of Adolescent Development

The prolific writings of Klein, Fairbairn, Winnicott, Guntrip, and Khan as well as those of other theorists, (Jacobson, P. Kernberg, Kohut, Mahler, Masterson, Rinsley, and Volkan) have all conveyed object relations insights about development which are relevant to adolescent psychology. Because of the far-reaching scope of these portraits of illness and development, I will briefly review the contributions of only a few of these theorists. By way of introduction to the chapters on object relations theories, my approach to this topic will be limited to Winnicott's, Fairbairn's and Khan's ideas about adolescence, and it will not include a comprehensive summary of object relations theories.

Object relations theorists have provided elaborations of the effects of human relationships on all aspects of development and psychopathology. In critical summaries of object relations theories, Greenberg and Mitchell (1983), Hamilton (1989) and Kwawer (1981) all credited the use of object relations concepts with facilitating the analyses of individuals with many forms of severe disorders. Although Klein (1935, 1946) wrote relatively little about adolescence, she ascertained that disturbances of late adolescence continued the anxieties of the paranoid-schizoid and depressive positions. The basis for a distinct object relations theory of adolescence was contained in Winnicott's concepts of ego relatedness and the facilitating environment. Winnicott (1971) attributed adolescents' psychic disturbances to environmental failures, more than to specific forms of character pathology. Klein, Winnicott and Fairbairn all held that, throughout development, character trends expressed internalizations of (and defenses against) ties to bad object attachments. Unlike Klein, Fairbairn and later Guntrip rejected both the death instinct's primacy, and drive theory, in favor of object seeking as the fundamental source of human motivation. Guntrip (1969, 1971) classified the inner sense of individuality, which blossomed during adolescence, as one of the personality's basic needs. Khan contributed to an object relations theory of adolescence by his descriptions of sexuality, and by his discussion of adolescents' identity disturbance.

In Khan's (1974, 1979) renewal of Winnicott's ideas, adolescents' lack of identity stemmed from disturbances in early body ego development and pathological identifications with the mother. Khan's view was that the latent emotionality of such early body ego experience found expression, during adulthood, in sexual intercourse and in the excitement of sexual perversions. Khan's discussions of his adolescent patients' affectivity elucidated Winnicott's use of countertransference with adolescents. According to each of these object relations theorists I have mentioned, the repetitive feelings inherent in internalized attachments persisted in their influence on defenses during the developmental predicaments of adolescence.

Winnicott (1958, 1965A, 1965B) linked ego relatedness, developmentally, with not only the baby's capacity to be alone, but also the baby's foundation of selfhood. The adolescent's relationship with the sexually maturing body reiterated this ego relatedness of mother-child body centered interactions. Winnicott's reports of his analytic work with adolescents kept in focus his objective of bolstering their development beyond the Oedipal level. This aim was achieved with a number of Winnicott's adolescent patients by his willingness to play and by his use of the squiggle game. Nevertheless, Winnicott's (1954A, 1954B, 1968) primary therapeutic goal with adolescents was always to make sure that the patient used the transference in order to overcome deprivations in maternal care.

Winnicott came to work with adolescent patients relatively late in his career as a psychoanalyst. His complex ideas on development seemed to include an apparent contradiction about the nature of adolescents' assertiveness or passivity in the emotional growth process. In agreement with Anna Freud, Winnicott (1971, 1975) speculated that adolescents' disturbances were often indistinguishable from the problems they encountered on the way to independence. He assigned to the analyst the crucial task of maintaining complete subservience to the traumas which the patient needed to stage. For Winnicott, narcissistic and borderline traits expressed adolescent patients' underlying core experiences of unreality and madness. His pronouncements about these ego states of unreality resembled the interpersonal theorists' accounts of disturbed youths' bouts of disintegration. With schizoid adolescents, Winnicott especially allowed the patient the crucial opportunity to unconsciously create the psychoanalyst. In his discussion of adolescent immaturity, Winnicott (1986) presented a hypothesis which outlined adolescents' essential involvement with the unconscious murder of their parents. This involvement was said to foster pubertal and postpubertal maturation. However, adolescents were depicted, elsewhere in Winnicott's writings, as fundamentally passive and reactive. Their psychic assertiveness was reduced to the passive status of remaining captive hostages of their peers and biological maturation. Winnicott designated adolescents' negotiation of developmental tasks as a process of waiting "in the doldrums".

The ideas of Winnicott and Fairbairn were only partially compatible with Freud's psychosexual theory and his views of adolescence. Winnicott's underscoring of adolescents' unconscious destructiveness suggested that he endorsed a Kleinian view of adolescence. This emphasis on adolescents' murderous fantasies raised the possibility that his developmental theory fell into the same conceptual trap of diminishing the importance of the real family, for which he had criticized Klein. However, Winnicott acknowledged elsewhere that analytic work with adolescents was ineffective without the presence of a healthy family which fostered maturation. These seemingly contradictory ideas about adolescent development did not culminate in a theory of adolescent character pathology which was as fully articulated as Winnicott's theories of infantile trauma. While Winnicott described the adolescent's inner reality, contemporary object relations theorists have delineated the dialectic process of introjection and projection during adolescence. Psychoanalytic family theorists, principally Shapiro, Zinner and colleagues (1975), have applied both object relations theory and systems theory to the exploration of family contributions to narcissistic and borderline adolescents' character trends. Object relations theories of adolescence have also been fully articulated by several contemporary authors. Included in this Volume are major theoretical papers by Lewis and Meltzer. Meltzer (1967) summarized the splitting processes that characterize the adolescent's shifting experience of identity, and Lewis (1987) traced impacted adolescent development to the remnants of the infantile paranoid-schizoid position.

SUMMARY

The foremost implication of the Freudian theories of adolescence has been that the analyst enters into an alliance with the patient's psychosexual development. During sessions, stock is routinely taken of the adolescent patient's defenses and drive fixations. The interpersonal and object relations theories of adolescents' character formation varied with each other and also with the assumptions of classical Freudian metapsychology. Yet, Sullivan, Fairbairn and Winnicott all stressed relatedness in character formation. They each urged that the attitudes of the actual person in significant relationships, as well as the internal representations of the self and the object, shaped the character tendencies of the child or adolescent. Sullivan was very outspoken about his belief that there could be no uniformly valid theory of character, because people are unique. However, for Sullivan, the needs for the validation of self worth, and for freedom from anxiety, were universal stimuli for the increasing organization of character trends. In both interpersonal theory and object relations theories dissociative processes were of paramount importance, as defensive operations. Dissociation, by the adolescent, resulted in further instances of ego splitting (for Fairbairn), of the not-me (for Sullivan), and of the false self (for Winnicott). Crucial also for the interpersonal and relational treatment models has been the analyst's role as an emotionally available, competent adult who uses immersion in the process to explicate the adolescent patient's failures to take advantage of developmental opportunities. In spite of their theoretical differences, Sullivan, Fairbairn, and Winnicott spoke with a singular voice in dismissing the exclusive significance of libidinal fixations in character consolidation.

Freud's Case of Dora and the Analytic Relationship with Adolescents

I now wish to discuss one aspect of Freud's case of Dora as an addendum to this short critical appraisal. The analysis of Dora readily lends itself to scrutiny of the confluence of the psychoanalytic models' clinical theories of adolescent analysis. Freud's (1905B) study of Dora has been one of his most widely cited and frequently criticized case monographs. As a result of this first analysis of an adolescent, Freud came to acknowledge and appreciate the importance of negative transference and resistance. So many theoretical papers have been written about Dora, that the limited scope of my objective will be to use the analysis of her first dream in order to contrast clinical implications of the Freudian, object relations and interpersonal theories of adolescence. This highly difficult case was not intended by Freud to be a treatise on psychoanalytic technique, and it introduced the complications imposed by his analytic work with adolescents. My specific aim in referring to Dora's first dream will be to compare the three developmental models' current outlooks on adolescents' psychopathology.

In a 1900 letter to Fliess, Freud (1950) first mentioned Dora as an adolescent patient whose analysis had opened smoothly, but the case study was not published until 1905. Dora had first consulted Freud when she was sixteen years old, and she later agreed to begin her analysis, when she was eighteen at the urging of her father who was one of Freud's former patients. Dora had left a suicide note which her parents found. At the start of her analysis, she reported numerous conversion symptoms, such as dizziness, headaches, aphonia, coughing and neuralgia. Dora's overall presentation was that of an hysteric. Freud's etiological explanation for her symptoms contained his axiom that hysterical symptoms represented repressed, conflictual fantasies of sexual activity. A later account of Dora indicated that her analysis did not result in either long lasting symptomatic relief or characterological change. Felix Deutsch (1957) briefly treated Dora as an adult. In a far from felicitous statement of her mental status, Deutsch reported a description of the forty year old Dora as a "most repulsive" hysteric. In Freud's (1905) postscript to the case, he determined that the treatment failure - Dora's abrupt termination - took place because of his failure to quickly interpret the Oedipal transference and his failure to recognize homosexual elements in the transference. A number of important essays about Dora have yielded alternate Freudian and interpersonal explanations for both her precipitous flight from therapy and its limited efficacy (Blos, 1972; Erikson, 1962; Kanzer, 1980; Glenn, 1980; Levenson, 1981; Muslin and Gill, 1978; Rogow, 1978).

Current assessments of Dora's personality might begin with the surface manifestations of her hysterical character style, namely her compensatory self-dramatization, her global, impressionistic thinking and the immersion of her conflicts and repressed emotionality in her conversion symptoms. From our contemporary perspective, these tendencies would be understood as defensive expressions of failures in adolescent development. They would likewise be seen as the result of the internalization of destructive patterns of family relationships which were unknowingly recreated in the analytic relationship. Further analysis might reveal Dora's longstanding anxieties and affective configurations involving betrayal, self-hatred, the fear of annihilation and unconscious surrender to the experience of exploitation. The transference-countertransference exchanges would need to be investigated along these dynamic lines by clinicians of each psychoanalytic orientation. The ensuing observations will follow the outline of Freudian, interpersonal and object relations responses to the clinical material. Dora's characterological and developmental problems were symbolized by the first dream she reported to Freud:

> A house was on fire. My father was standing beside my bed and woke me up. I dressed quickly. Mother wanted to stop and save her jewel case, but father said: "I refuse to let myself and my two children be burnt for the sake of your jewel case". (Freud, 1905B, p.64)

The essence of the dream was interpreted to be Dora's repudiation of repressed sexual excitement at being kissed by her father's friend, Herr K. Herr K. had tried to seduce Dora when she was fourteen. The dream was a recurrent one which began when Dora was sixteen, after Herr K. proposed to her, and she felt indignant and frightened of further seduction.

In addition, Dora's attacks of hysterical coughing and nervous asthma were considered by Freud to be both the result of sexual guilt and the equivalent of an unconscious fellatio fantasy. This fantasy was said to represent Dora's wish for sexual contact with her father, by means of identifying herself with Frau K. with whom her father had a longstanding affair. Dora's unconscious sexual longings for Herr K., and for her father, as well as her repressed homosexual feelings were depicted as the basis for the atmosphere of psychic danger which pervaded the dream. Freud did not connect the dream either with Dora's suicide note, which had first brought her to treatment, or with her likely feelings of betrayal, self-hatred and abandonment. His deduction was that Dora's clinical symptomatology emerged from her hysterical renunciation of the seducer, her own sexual excitation, and her repressed Oedipal wishes. Such factors as the parents' hypocrisy, the 19th century Viennese cultural attitudes towards women, and the influence of unrecognized countertransference hostility were beyond the realm of Freud's analysis of the transference and resistance. Dora's feelings of outrage and her provocativeness were no doubt fueled by her lack of individuation and her surreptitious betrayal by both of her parents. Dora had been betrayed by her parents' disbelief of her account of Herr K.'s sexual advances. Neither parent acknowledged Dora's father's offering her to Herr K., as compensation for his own affair with Frau K. Freud recognized, but made no mention of, the impact on Dora of the family's pretense and hypocrisy. If the reproach in the dream referred to Dora's feelings in addition to those of her father, then it signified her anger at her father's manipulativeness and dishonesty. The reproach in the dream simultaneously conveyed an attack on Freud, for his exposure of Dora's sexual secrets, at the expense of not validating her potentially painful insights into the family secrets. According to Freud's dream theory, the ties between manifest dream symbols and unconscious sexual wishes were repressed, because of the dangers of childhood sexual impulses and moral inhibitions. Dora's anxiety, and fury, about the possibility of betrayal and in authenticity in the transference-countertransference might have also been repressed.

Dora's dream took place following Freud's interpretative statements about her autoerotic stimulation. Dora may have thus needed to retaliate for the frustration of her wish for validation, and encouragement, to use both herself, and the transference, in order to overcome her self-destructiveness and her attention seeking conversion symptoms. The dramatic presentation of Dora's father, as the heroic rescuer in the dream, hinted at Dora's ambivalence about an idealized father, as well as the provocativeness and narcissism which were presented to her as a model for identification. Finally, the father's appearance, in the dream, at the undressed Dora's bedside in the (passionate) heat of the fire pointed to Herr K's attempts at seduction as well as her feelings of Oedipal betrayal.

Present day Freudian analysts would examine the effects of the family hypocrisy and enmeshment on Dora's unconscious fantasies, in addition to the links between her somatic symptoms and the feelings in her internalized relationships. Dora's ego ideal, her sense of identity, her problems with individuation and deidealization, her unconscious need to mother her own body, and the secondary gains of her remaining the Oedipal child would all be investigated. Anna Freud (1980) believed that the key to forming a therapeutic alliance with adolescent patients lay in helping the adolescent come to terms with the presence of some painful inner state which the analysis would address. Muslin and Gill (1978) pointed out that Freud's countertransference responses repeatedly interfered with his seeing transference references throughout the analysis. Blos (1972) formulated a number of criticisms of Freud's interpretations of Dora's sexual wishes. He indicated that Dora's incipient neurotic character was crystallized by the analysis which treated her as though she were an adult who had achieved psychic separation from the family. In an observation with which most psychoanalysts would agree, Blos argued that poorly timed id interpretations will be heard by adolescents as parental seductions.

Freud's interpretations about Dora's masturbatory conflicts, and her repressed wishes for sexual contact with both himself and her father, could have been heard as a seductive enticement. In a final criticism of Freud's handling of Dora, Erikson (1962) distinguished the role of psychological reality from the importance of historical actuality. Freud dismissed both the seriousness of Dora's interest in analysis and her request for validation of her perceptions. For Erikson, Freud's double failure consisted of his ignoring Dora's developmental considerations, and his not understanding that adolescent patients genuinely need validation of historical actuality.

Interpersonal and Object Relations
Aspects of Dora

From Sullivan's point of view, an adolescent patient, like Dora, would have needed to give up private disordered experience, during analysis, by making use of consensual validation. On the basis of the analyst's participant observation, the therapeutic cure for adolescents occurred through the elimination of dissociation and the newfound possibility of profiting from present and future life experience. As a telling comment on Erikson's comment, Levenson (1981) called into question Freud's assumption that patients' fantasies constituted the primary data of psychoanalytic inquiry. In interpersonal theory, transference-countertransference transactions have long been considered to be a continuous process of mutual influence. Freud's neglect of Dora's seduction by her family, and his overall neglect of other interpersonal issues, has been scrutinized by Slipp (1977), Spiegel (1977), and other authors.

Speculation about the origins of Freud's negative countertransference with Dora has in no way detracted from the momentous historical value of this fragmentary analysis. Gay's (1988) authoritative biography of Freud implied that several key relationships in Freud's life might have united the disparate elements of his countertransference feelings towards his female patients. Gay hypothesized that the adolescent Freud's unrequited love for his friend's sister, Gisela Fluss, unleashed highly impassioned psychic forces. In addition, Freud's emotional over involvement with his oldest daughter was reported, by Gay, to have, on occasion, reached an extreme intensity. At the time of Dora's analytic sessions with Freud, in 1900, Anna Freud would have been approximately five years old and in the throes of the Oedipal conflict. Rogow (1978) believed that Dora was really Ida Bauer, the sister of a well known Marxist, socialist Austrian political leader. However, Kanzer's (1980) investigative efforts yielded the conclusion that Dora's real name was Rosa, the name of Freud's most cherished sister, and also the name of his sister's nursemaid. If Freud unconsciously identified Dora with any of these women, then Dora's analysis might have assembled his detachment and his hostility as defenses against his own unresolved Oedipal longings. With the transposition of Dora's analysis to the present, the analyst would not be exempt from considering all   potential sources of countertransference influence on resistance and transference. A contemporary interpersonal analysis of Dora's dream would thus include Dora's possible awareness of her father's duplicity and seductiveness, as well as her recognition of, and contribution to, Freud's unwitting re-creation of her father's condescending rejection.

From an interpersonal, relational point of view, Dora's first dream offered glimpses of her deepest, most profound anxieties about annihilation and destructiveness in relationships. According to Kleinian theory, Dora's masturbation fantasies could not have escaped either the powerful influence of the death instinct, or her infantile conflicts with part-objects. These fantasies would be heard as an arena for her bellicose impulses and anxieties. If Dora associated the jewel case in the dream with her mother and herself, rather than her genitals, then the dream might have expressed the death anxiety which was connected with her fear of separation and her wish for the internalized good mother. Dora's repressed masturbation fantasies and sexual wishes could have therefore suggested a retreat from her terror of individuation, as well as the fear of her own rage projected onto the devouring penis and the annihilating breast. Furthermore, if Freud identified Dora with his sister's servant, then this dream might have also expressed the enactment of his wish to be served and her unconscious self image of being submissive to exploitation. A contemporary analysis of Dora would necessitate her experiencing and relinquishing the affective connections between the frantic, devalued, victimized self and the object as the seductive, hostile agent of betrayal. From an interpersonal perspective, these affective connections represent crucial relational patterns that would be recreated in analyst - patient interactions.

In his extension of Klein's ideas, Fairbairn accounted for hysterical character trends, like Dora's, as recreations in the genital sphere of earlier oral problems. He maintained that Freud's polarization of libido and aggression was a false dichotomy, because feelings of hate lay in readiness beneath all intense dysphoric emotions. According to Winnicott's terminology, an adolescent analysand, like Dora, would need to ruthlessly demand a new maternal object in order to fully prosper in relating. At the very least, Dora would be presented with the ambience of, what Winnicott considered to be an optimal environment for facilitating her genuine self's return, from dissociation. What would have been of great concern (for Fairbairn) was the absorption of Dora's wish for her father's penis into her need for his emotional availability, and (for Sullivan) the effect of this unsatisfied need on Dora's self-esteem and interpersonal inference making. Present day analysts, of all orientations, might investigate Dora's relationship with her body as a vehicle for her object relationships, her tentative autonomy, her internalized rage and her other dissociated affects. In partial accordance with the current Freudian and interpersonal models of clinical practice, an object relations approach to Dora's dreams would use the transference-countertransference transactions as a potential source of understanding of both her developmental conflicts and the therapeutic interaction.

CONCLUSION

The Freudian, interpersonal and object relations developmental theories have suggested different starting points for the analytic investigation of adolescents' characterological problems. Each of these three theoretical models have established the conceptual connections between problems in adolescent development and the emergence of psychopathology, but they have done so from different directions. Freudian theorists emphasize the integration of the drives and defenses in the libidinal fixations and the structural changes of adolescence. While interpersonal theorists stress dissociative processes and familial forces in self-alienation, in Sullivan's pragmatic vision of personality maturation, the self system, which includes character, reduces the adolescent to a diminished caricature of what he or she might have become. Object relations theories highlight disruptive developmental anxieties inherent in adolescents' self-object dialogues. In Winnicott's optimistic theory of development, some degree of insanity is necessary for the adolescent's optimal adjustment. Winnicott claims that this measure of madness is essential if the adolescent is to avoid sacrificing individuality in light of the need to remain unknown, by adults, yet authentically alive. Developmental approaches to adolescents' psychopathology, such as Esman's (1985) treatment philosophy carefully detailed in Section III, are at least partially compatible with clinical work from the perspective of each of the analytic orientations.

REFERENCES

Aichhorn, A. (1935), Some causes of delinquency *Wayward Youth*. New York: Viking Press.

Anthony, E.J. (1976) Between yes and no: The potentially neutral area where the adolescent and his therapist can meet. *Adolescent Psychiatry*, 3, 323-344.

Barnett, J. (1978A), Insight and therapeutic change. *Contemporary Psychoanalysis*, 14, 534-544.

Barnett, J. (1978B), On the dynamics of interpersonal isolation. *Journal of the American Academy of Psychoanalysis*, 6, 59-70.

Barnett, J. (1980), Self and character. *Journal of the American Academy of Psychoanalysis*, 8, 337-352.

Bilmes, M. (1967) Shame and delinquency. *Contemporary Psychoanalysis*, 3, 113-133.

Blos, P. (1962), *On Adolescence: A Psychoanalytic Interpretation*. Glencoe: Free Press.

Blos, P. (1967), The second individuation process of adolescence. *Psychoanalytic Study of the Child*, 22, 162-186.

Blos, P. (1968), Character formation in adolescence. *Psychoanalytic Study of the Child*, 23, 245-263.

Blos, P. (1971), Adolescent concretization: A contribution to the theory of delinquency. In: I. Marcus, (Ed.) *Currents in Psychoanalysis*. New York: International Universities Press.

Blos, P. (1972), The epigenesis of the adult neurosis. *Psychoanalytic Study of the Child*, 27, 106-135.

Blos, P. (1977), When and how does adolescence end: Structural criteria for adolescence closure. *Adolescent Psychiatry*, 5, 5-17.

Blos, P. (1980), The life cycle as indicated by the nature of the transference in the psychoanalysis of adolescents. *International Journal of Psychoanalysis*, 61, 145-151.

Deutsch, F. (1957), A footnote to Freud's "Fragment of an analysis of a case of hysteria". In: On the Mysterious Leap from the Mind to the Body. New York: International Universities Press.

Ekstein, R. (1971), Psychotic adolescents and their quest for goals. In: *The Challenge: Despair and Hope in the Conquest of Inner Space*. New York:Brunner Mazel.

Erikson, E. (1956), The problem of ego identity. *Journal of the American Psychoanalytic Association*, 4, 56-121.

Erikson, E. (1959A), *Identity and the Life Cycle*. New York: International Universities Press.

Erikson, E. (1959B), Late adolescence. In: E. Schlein (Ed.) *A Way of Looking at things: Selected Papers of Erik Erikson From 1930 - 1980*. New York: Norton: 1987.

Erikson, E. (1962), Reality and actuality. *Journal of the American Psychoanalytic Association*, 10, 451-474.

Erikson, E. (1968A), *Identity, Youth and Crisis*. New York: Norton.

Erikson, E. (1968B), Psychosocial Identity. In: E. Schlein (Ed.) *A Way of Looking at things: Selected Papers of Erik Erikson 1930- 1980. New York: Norton, 1987.*

Esman, A. (1980), Midadolescence - Foundations for later psychopathology. In: S. Greenspan & G. Pollack's (Eds.) *The Course of Life: Psychoanalytic Contributions Toward Understanding Personality Development. Volume II:Latency, Adolescence, and Youth, 419-430. Washington, D.C.: NIMH.*

Esman, A. (1985). A developmental approach to the psychotherapy of adolescents. *Adolescent Psychiatry*, 12, 119-133.

Fairbairn, W. (1952), *Psychoanalytic Studies of the Personality*, London: Tavistock.

Fairbairn, W. (1954), Observations on the nature of hysterical states. *British Journal of Medical Psychology*, 27, 105-125.

Freud, A. (1937), The Ego and the Mechanisms of Defense. New York: International Universities.

Freud, A. (1958), Adolescence. *Psychoanalytic Study of the Child.* 13:255-278.

Freud, A. (1965), Normality and Pathology in Childhood. New York: International Universities Press.

Freud, A. (1980), Treatment alliance. In: J. Sandler, H. Kennedy, and R. Tyson (Eds.), *The Technique of Child Psychoanalysis: Discussions with Anna Freud.* Cambridge: Harvard University Press.

Freud, S. (1905a), Three essays on the theory of sexuality. *The Standard Edition of the Complete Psychological Works of Sigmund Freud,* 7:125-245. London: Hogarth Press.

Freud, S. (1905b), Fragment for analysis for a case of hysteria. *The Standard Edition of the Complete Psychological Works of Sigmund Freud,* 7:1-122. London: Hogarth Press.

Freud, S. (1950), Extracts from the Fliess papers. *The Standard Edition of the Complete Psychological Works of Sigmund Freud,* 1:173-280. London:Hogarth Press.

Fromm, E. (1941), *Escape From Freedom.* New York: Holt, Rinehart and Winston.

Fromm, E. (1947), *Man For Himself.* New York: Holt, Rinehart and Winston.

Gay, P. (1988), *Freud: A Life for Our Time.* New York: Norton.

Giovacchini, P. (1975), Productive procrastination: Technical factors in the treatment of the adolescent. *Adolescent Psychiatry,* 4, 352-370.

Glenn, J. (1980), Freud's adolescent patients: Katarina, Dora, and the "homosexual woman". In: Kanzer, M. & Glenn, J. (Eds.) *Freud and His Patients.* New York: Aronson.

Greenberg, J., and Mitchell, S. (1983), *Object Relations in Psychoanalytic Theory.* Cambridge: Harvard University Press.

Grinberg, L. Grinberg, R. (1974), Pathological aspects of identity in adolescence. *Contemporary Psychoanalysis,* 10, 27-40.

Guntrip, H. (1961), *Personality Structure and Human Interaction: The Developing Synthesis of Psychodynamic Theory.* London: Hogarth Press.

Guntrip, H. (1969), *Schizoid Phenomena, Object Relations and the Self.* London: Hogarth Press.

Guntrip, H. (1971), *Psychodynamic Theory, Therapy and the Self.* New York: Basic Books.

Hamilton, N. (1989), A critical review of object relations theory. *American Journal of Psychiatry*, 146, 1552-1560.

Horney, K. (1937), *The Neurotic Personality of Our Time.* New York: Norton.

Horney, K. (1939), *New Ways in Psychoanalysis.* New York: Norton.

Horney, K. (1951), *Neurosis and Human Growth.* New York: Norton.

Jones, E. (1922), Some problems of adolescence. In: *Papers on Psychoanalysis.* London: Balliere, Tindall, & Cox, 1948.

Josselson, R. (1987), Identity diffusion: A long term follow up. *Adolescent Psychiatry*, 14, 230-258.

Kanzer, M. (1980), Dora's imagery: The flight from a burning house. In: Kanzer, M. & J. Glenn, J. (Eds.) *Freud and His Patients.* New York:Aronson.

Kasin, E. (1971). Youth in turmoil. *Contemporary Psychoanalysis*, 8, 48-60.

Kernberg, O. (1976), *Object Relations Theory and Clinical Psychoanalysis.* New York: Aronson.

Kernberg, P. (1979), Psychoanalytic profile of the borderline adolescent. *Adolescent Psychiatry*, 7, 234-256.

Khan, M. (1974), Silence as communication. In: *The Privacy of the Self.* New York: International Universities Press.

Khan, M. (1979), *Alienation in Perversions.* New York: International Universities Press.

Klein, M. (1935), A contribution to the psychoanalysis of manic depressive states. In: *Contributions to Psychoanalysis, 1921-1945.* New York: McGraw Hill, 1964.

Klein, M. (1946), Notes on some schizoid mechanisms. In: *Envy, Gratitude, and Other Works*, 1946-1963, New York: Delacorte Press, 1975.

Kwawer, J. (1981), Object relations and interpersonal theories. *Contemporary Psychoanalysis*, 17, 276-289.

Laufer, M. (1968), The body image, the function of masturbation and adolescence: Problems of the ownership of the body. *Psychoanalytic Study of the Child*, 23, 114-137.

Laufer, M. (1981), Adolescent breakdown and the transference neurosis. *International Journal of Psychoanalysis*, 62, 51-59.

Laufer, M. & Laufer, E. (1984), *Adolescence and Developmental*

Breakdown. New Haven: Yale University Press.

Levenson, E. (1981), Facts or fantasies. On the nature of psychoanalytic data. *Contemporary Psychoanalysis,* 17:486-500.

Levenson, E., Stockhamer, N., and Feiner, A. (1967), Family transactions in the etiology of dropping out of college. *Contemporary Psychoanalysis,* 3, 134-152.

Lewis, O. (1987), The paranoid-schizoid position and pathologic regression in early adolescence. *Journal of the American Academy of Psychoanalysis,* 15, 503-519,.

Masterson, J. (1967), *The Psychiatric Dilemma of Adolescence: A Developmental approach.* Boston: Little Brown. New York: John Wiley & Sons.

Masterson, J. (1974), Intensive psychotherapy of the adolescent with a borderline syndrome. In: S. Arieti (Ed.), *American Handbook of Psychiatry. Volume 2.* New York: Basic Books.

Masterson, J. (1978), The borderline adolescent: An object relations view. *Adolescent Psychiatry,* 6, 344-359.

Meltzer, D. (1967), Identification and socialization in adolescents. *Contemporary Psychoanalysis,* 3, 96-103.

Mitchell, S. (1988), *Relational Concepts in Psychoanalysis.* Cambridge: Harvard University Press.

Muslin, H. & Gill, M. (1978), Transference in the Dora case. *Journal of the American Psychoanalytic Association,* 36, 311-328.

Redl, F. And Wineman, D. (1951), *Children Who Hate.* New York:Free Press.

Ritvo, S. (1971), Late adolescence:Developmental and clinical considerations. *Psychoanalytic Study of the Child,* 26, 241-263.

Rogow, W. (1978), A further footnote to Freud's "Fragment of an analysis of a case of hysteria". *Journal of the American Psychoanalytic Association,* 29, 331-376.

Sandler, J. (1981), Character traits and object relationships. *Psychoanalytic Quarterly,* 50, 694-708.

Shapiro, E., Zinner, J., Shapiro, R. and Berkowitz, D. (1975), The influence of family experience on borderline personality development. International Review of Psychoanalysis, 2, 399-411.

Singer, E. (1965), *Key Concepts in Psychotherapy.* New York: Basic Books.

Slipp, S. (1977), Interpersonal factors in hysteria. *Journal of the*

28

American Academy of Psychoanalysis, 5, 359-376.

Spiegel, R. (1977), Freud and the women in his world. *Journal of the American Academy of Psychoanalysis, 5, 377-402.*

Sullivan, H. (1940), *Conceptions of Modern Psychiatry.* New York: Norton.

Sullivan, H. (1953), *The Interpersonal Theory of Psychiatry.* New York: Norton.

Thompson, C. (1964), Psychopathology in *adolescence. In: M. Green (Ed.) Interpersonal Psychoanalysis, New York: Basic Books.*

Wallerstein, R. (1998), Erikson's concept of ego identity reconsidered. *Journal of the American Psychoanalytic Association, 46, 229-247.*

Winnicott, D. (1954A), Metapsychological and clinical aspects of regression within the psychoanalytic setup. In: *Through Paediatrics to Psychoanalysis: Collected Papers.* London: Hogarth Press, 1975.

Winnicott, D. (1954B), Withdrawal and regression. In: *Through Pediatrics to Psychoanalysis: Collected Papers.* London: Hogarth Press, 1975.

Winnicott, D. (1965a), *The Maturational Processes and the Facilitating Environment.* London: Hogarth Press, 1965.

Winnicott, D. (1965b), Adolescence: Struggling through the doldrums. In: *The Family and Individual Development.* London: Tavistock Publications, 1965.

Winnicott, E. (1968), Adolescent immaturity. In: C. Winnicott, R. Shepherd, & M. Davis (Eds.) *Home Is Where We Start From: Essays by a Psychoanalyst.* New York: Norton, 1986.

Winnicott, D. (1971), *Playing and Reality.* New York:BasicBooks.

Winnicott, D. (1975), *Through Pediatrics to Psychoanalysis: Collected Papers.* London: Hogarth Press.

Wolf, E. (1982), Adolescence: Psychology of the self and self objects. *Adolescent Psychiatry, 12, 171-181.*

CHAPTER TWO
ADOLESCENCE[1]

Anna Freud

I. Adolescence in the Psychoanalytic Theory
Introduction

I return to the subject of adolescence after an interval of twenty two years. During this time much has happened in analytic work to throw added light on the problems concerned and to influence the conditions of life for young people, whether normal or abnormal. Nevertheless, in spite of partial advances, the position with regard to the analytic study of adolescence is not a happy one, and especially unsatisfactory when compared with that of early childhood. With the latter period, we feel sure of our ground, and in possession of a wealth of material and information which enables us to assume authority and apply analytic findings to practical problems of upbringing. When it comes to adolescence, we feel hesitant and, accordingly, cannot satisfy the parents or educational workers who apply for help to us and to our knowledge. One can hear it said frequently that adolescence is a neglected period, a stepchild where analytic thinking is concerned.

These complaints, which come from two sides, from the parents as well as from the analytic workers themselves, seem to me to warrant closer study and investigation than the have received so far.

Adolescence in the Psychoanalytic Literature

The psychoanalytic study of adolescence began, as is well known in 1905 with the relevant chapter of the *Three Essays on Sexuality*. Here, puberty was described as the time when the changes set in which give infantile sexual life its final shape. Subordination of the erotogenic zones to the primacy of the genital zone; the setting up of new sexual aims, different for males and females; and the finding of new sexual objects outside the family were listed as the main events. While this exposition explained many features of the adolescent process and behavior which had been unexplained before, the newly developed notion of the existence of an infantile sexual life could not but lower the significance of adolescence in the eyes of the

---

[1] The content of this paper is based on material collected in the Hempstead Child Therapy Clinic...

investigators. Before the publication of the *Three Essays*, adolescence had derived major significance form its role as the beginning of sex life in the individual; after the discovery of an infantile sex life, the status of adolescence was reduced to that of a period of final transformations, a transition and bridge between the diffuse infantile and genitally centered adult sexuality.

Seventeen years later, in 1922, Ernest Jones, London, published a paper on "Some Problems of Adolescence" which dwelt on a "correlation between adolescence and infancy" as its most distinctive point. Following the pronouncement in the *Three Essays* that the phase of development corresponding to the period between the ages of two and five must be regarded as an important precursor of the subsequent final organization, he showed in detail how the "the individual recapitulates and expands in the second decennium of life the development he passed through during the first five years..." (p. 398). He ascribed the difference in "the circumstances in which the development takes place" but went as far as propounding "the general law... that adolescence recapitulates infancy, and that the precise way in which a given person   will pass through the necessary stages of development in adolescence is to a very great extent determined by the form of his infantile development" (p. 399). In short: "these stages are passed through are on different planes at the two periods of infancy and adolescence, but in very similar ways in the same individual" (p. 399).

Jones's important but isolated contribution to the problem coincided with a peak in the publications of Seigfried Bernfeld in Vienna, a true explorer of youth, who combined work as a clinical analyst and teacher of analysis with the unceasing study of adolescence in all its aspect of individual and group behavior, reaction to social influences, sublimations, etc. His most significant addition to the analytic theory was the description of a specific kind of male adolescent development (1923), the so-called "protracted" type which extends far beyond the time limit normal for adolescent characteristics, and is conspicuous by "tendencies toward productivity whether artistic, literary or scientific, and by a strong bend toward idealistic aims and spiritual values...." As the solid background for his assumptions, Bernfeld published, in cooperation with W. Hoffer, a wealth of material consisting of self observations of adolescents, their diaries, poetic productions, etc.

While Bernfeld accounted in this manner for the elaborations of the normal adolescent processes by the impact of internal frustrations and external, environmental pressures, August Aichhorn, also in Vienna, approached the problem from the angle of dissocial and criminal development. His work lay with those young people who answer to the same pressures with failure to adapt, faulty superego development and revolt against the community. His book *Wayward Youth (1925)* acquired world renown as the outstanding pioneering attempt to carry psychoanalytic knowledge into the difficult realm of the problems of the young offender.

Based on familiarity with S. Bernfeld's views, and intimately connected with A. Aichhorn's studies, I contributed in 1936 two papers under the titles "The Ego and the Id at Puberty" and "Instinctual Anxiety During Puberty." In my case, interest in the adolescent problems was derived from my concern with the struggles of the ego to master the tensions and pressures arising from the drive derivatives, struggles which lead in the normal case to character formation, in their pathological outcome to the formation of neurotic symptoms. I described this battle between ego and id as terminated by a first truce at the beginning of the latency period and breaking out once more with the first approach to puberty, when the distribution of forces inside the individual is upset by quantitative and qualitative changes in the drives. Threatened with anxiety by the drive development, the ego, as it has been formed in childhood enters into a struggle for survival in which all the available methods of defense are brought into play and strained to the utmost. The results, that is the personality changes which are achieved, vary. Normally, the organization of the ego and superego alter sufficiently to accommodate the new, mature forms of sexuality. In less favorable instances a rigid, immature ego succeeds in inhibiting or distorting sexual maturity; in some cases the id impulses succeed in creating utter confusion and chaos in what has been an orderly, socially directed ego during the latency period. I made the point that, more than any other time of life, adolescence with its typical conflicts provides the analyst with instructive pictures of the interplay and sequence of internal danger, anxiety, defense activity, transitory or permanent symptom formation, and mental breakdown.

Interest increased in the post war years and brought a multitude of contributions, especially from the United States. Fortunately for the student of the subject, Leo A. Spiegel published in 1951 a lengthy "Review of Contributions to a Psychoanalytic Theory of Adolescence." Although his attempt to construct an integrated theory out of widely divergent parts could hardly be successful, the paper serves a most useful purpose by abstracting, reviewing and classifying the material. He grouped the publications under headings such as:

"Classification of Phenomenology" (Bernfeld, Hartmann, Kris, and Lowenstien, Wittels)
"Object Relations" (Bernfeld, Buxbaum, H. Deutsch, Erikson, Fenichel, A. Freud, W. Hoffer, Jones, A. Katan-Angel, Landauer)
"Defense Mechanism" (Bernfeld, H. Deutsch, Fenichel, A. Freud, Greenacre, E. Kris) "Creativity" (Bernfeld, A. Freud)
"Sexual Activity" (Balint, Bernfeld, Buxbaumn, H. Deutsch, Federn, Ferenczi, S. Freud, Lampl-de Groot)
"Aspects of Ego Functioning" (Fenichel, A. Freud, Harnik, Hoffer, Landauer)
"Treatment" (Aichhorn, K. R. Eissler, A. Freud, Gitelson, A. Katan, M.Klein, Laundauer, A.Reich).

A detailed bibliography attached to the review contained altogether forty-one papers by thirty-four authors, covering apparently every theoretical, clinical, and technical aspect of the subject.

But in spite of this impressive list of contributors and contributions the dissatisfaction with our knowledge of the field remained unaltered, nor did our own, or the parents', confidence in our analytic skill with adolescent patients increase. There was now much published evidence to the contrary; nevertheless, adolescence remained, as it had been before, a stepchild in psychoanalytic theory.

Some Difficulties of Fact-Finding Concerning Adolescence

There are, I believe, two different causes, which may, possibly, account for our bewilderment when faced with all the intricacies of the adolescent process.

When, in our capacity as analysts, we investigate mental states, we rely, basically, on two methods: either on the analysis of individuals in whom that particular state of mind is in action at the moment, or on the reconstruction of that state in analytic treatment undertaken at a later date. The results of these two procedures, used either singly, or in combination with each other, have taught us all that we, as analysts, know about the developmental stages of the human mind.[2]
It happens that these two procedures, which have served us well for all other periods of life, prove less satisfactory and less productive of results when applied to adolescent.

(I) Reconstruction of adolescence in adult analysis.- As regards reconstruction, I am impressed how seldom in the treatment of my adult cases I succeed in reviving their adolescent experiences in full force. By that I do not mean to imply that adult patients have an amnesia for their adolescence which resembles in extent or in depth the amnesia for their early childhood. On the contrary, the memories of the events of the adolescent period are, normally, retained in consciousness and told to the analyst without apparent difficulty.   Masturbation in preadolescence and adolescence, the first moves toward intercourse, etc., may even play a dominant part in the patient's conscious memories and, as we know well, are made use of to overlay and hide the repressed masturbation conflicts and the buried sexual activities of early childhood. Further, in the analyses of sexually inhibited men who deplore the loss of erective potency, it is fairly easy to recover the memories of the bodily practices carried out in adolescence-frequently very crude and cruel ones-which served them at that time to prevent erections, or to suppress them as soon as they occurred. On the other hand, these memories contain no more than the bare facts, happenings and actions, divorced from the affects that accompanied them at the time. What we fail to recover, as a rule, is the atmosphere in which the adolescent lives, his anxieties, the height of elation or depth of despair, the quickly rising enthusiasms, the utter hopelessness, the burning-or at other times sterile-intellectual and philosophical preoccupations, the yearning for freedom, the sense of loneliness, the feeling of oppression by the parents, the impotent rages or hates directed against the adult world, the erotic crushes-whether homosexually or heterosexually directed-the suicidal fantasies, etc. These are elusive mood swings, difficult to revive which, unlike the affective states of infancy and early childhood, seem disinclined to re-emerge and be relived in connection with the person of the analyst. If this impression, which I gathered from my own cases, should be confirmed by other analysts of adults, such a failure- or partial failure- to reconstruct adolescence might account for some of the gaps in our appraisal of the mental processes during the period.

(ii) *Analysis during adolescence-* When discussing in his "Review" the contributions dealing with analytic therapy, Spiegel (1951) deplored what seemed to him an undue pessimism on the part of some authors. He pointed

[2] It may be worth while to remind the reader in this connection that our knowledge of the mental processes of infancy has been derived from reconstructions in the analyses of adults and was merely confirmed and enlarged later on by analyses or observations carried out in childhood.

to the need for adapting the analytic technique to the adolescent patients' particular situation and expressed surprise at the absence of explicit discussions of an introductory phase "analogous to the one used with children and delinquents."

Actually, since 1951, some further papers on the subject of technique appeared in print. Two of them dealt with the opening phase, (Fraiberg, 1955), (Noshpitz, 1957), a third with the terminal one (Adatto, 1958).

While these authors brought material to highlight the special technical difficulties encountered in the beginning and ending of therapy, work on adolescents done in our Hempstead Child Therapy Clinic emphasized special technical difficulties met with in the very center of it, i.e., at the critical moment when preadolescence gives way to adolescence proper, when the revolt against the parents is anticipated in the transference and tends to lead to a break with the analyst, i.e., to abrupt and undesirable termination of treatment from the patient's side.

Thus, according to experience, special difficulties are encountered in the beginning, in the middle, and in connection with the end of treatment. Put in other words, this can only mean that the analytic treatment of adolescents is a hazardous venture from beginning to end, a venture in which the analyst has to meet resistances of unusual strength and density. This is borne out by the comparison of adolescent with adult cases. In adult analysis we are used to handle the difficult technical situations with certain hysterical patients who cannot bear frustration in the transference and try to force the analyst to enact with them their revived love and hate feelings in an actual personal relationship. We are used to guard against the obsessional patients' technique of isolating words from affect and of tempting us to interpret unconscious content while it is divorced from its emotional cathexis. We attempt to deal with the narcissistic withdrawal of the borderline schizophrenics, the projections of the paranoid patents who turn their analyst into the persecuting enemy, the destructive hopelessness of the depressed who claim disbelief in any positive outcome of the analytic effort; the acting-out tendencies and the lack of insight of the delinquent or psychopathic characters. But in the disturbances named above, we meet either the one or the other of these technical difficulties, and we can adapt the analytic technique to the resistance which is specific for the type of mental disorder. Not so in adolescence where the patient may change rapidly from one of these emotional positions to the next, exhibit them all simultaneously, or in quick succession, leaving the analyst little time and scope to marshal his forces and change his handling of the case according to the changing need. *(iii)Obstacles in the libido economy. Comparison with the states of mourning and unhappy love*.- Experience has taught us that to take a serious view of such major and repeated inadequacies of the analytic technique. They cannot be explained away by individual characteristics of the patients under treatment nor by any accidental or environmental factors which run counter to it. nor can they be overcome simply by increased effort, skill and tact on the part of the analyst. They have to be taken as indications that something in the inner structure of the disturbances themselves differs markedly from the pattern of those illnesses for which the analytic technique has been devised originally and to which it is most frequently applied (Eissler, 1950). We have to gain insight into these divergences of pathology before we are in a position to revise our technique. Where the analyses of children, of delinquents and of certain borderline states are concerned, this has happened already. What the analytic technique had to provide for in these cases were the immaturity and weakness of the patients' ego; their lower threshold for the toleration of frustration; and the lesser importance of verbalization with increased importance of action (acting out) for their mental economy. It remains to be pointed out what corresponding factors are characteristic for the adolescent disorders, i.e., to what specific inner situation of the patients our technique has to be adjusted to make adolescents more amenable to analytic treatment.

So far as I am concerned, I am impressed by a similarity between the responses of these young patients and those of two other well known types of mental upset, namely the reactions to treatment during unhappy love affairs and during periods of mourning. In both these later states there is much mental suffering and, as a rule, the urgent wish to be helped; in spite of this, neither state answers well to analytic therapy. Our theoretical explanation of this comparative intractability is the is the following: being in love as well as mourning are emotional states in which the individual's libido is engaged fully in relation to a real love object of the present, or of the most recent past, the mental pain being caused by the difficult task to withdraw cathexis and give up a position which holds out no further hope for return of love, that is for satisfaction. While the individual is engaged in this struggle, insufficient libido is available to cathect the person of the analyst, or to flow back regressively and to reinvest former objects and positions. Consequently, neither the transference events nor the past become meaningful enough to yield material for interpretation. The immediate past (of love or of mourning) has to be given up before analytic therapy can become effective.

To my mind the libidinal position of the adolescent has much in common with the two states described above. The adolescent too is much engaged in an emotional struggle, and moreover in one of extreme urgency and immediacy. His libido is on the point of detaching itself from the parents and of cathecting new objects. Some mourning for the objects of the past is inevitable; so are the "crushes," i.e., the happy or unhappy love affairs with adults outside the family, or with other adolescents, whether of the opposite or of the same sex; so is, further, a certain amount of narcissistic withdrawal which bridges the gap during periods when no external object is cathected. Whatever the libidinal solution at a given moment may be, it will always be a preoccupation with the present time and, as described above, with little or no libido left available for investment either in the past or in the analyst.

If this supposition as to the libido distribution in the adolescent personality can be accepted as a correct statement, it can serve to explain some of our young patients' behavior in treatment, such as: their reluctance to cooperate; their lack of involvement in the therapy or in the relationship to the analyst; their battles for the reduction of weekly sessions; their unpunctuality; their missing of treatment sessions for the sake of outside activities; their sudden breaking off of treatment altogether. We learn here by contrast how much the continuity of the average adult analysis owes to the fact of the analyst being a highly cathected object, quite apart from the essential role played by the transference in the production of material.

There are, of course, those cases where the analyst himself becomes the new love object of the adolescent, i.e., the object of the "crush", a constellation which will heighten the young patient's keenness to be "treated." But apart from improved attendance and punctuality, this may mean merely that the analyst is brought against another of the specific difficulties of the analyses of adolescents, namely the urgency of their needs, their intolerance for frustration and their tendency to treat whatever relationship evolves as a vehicle for wish fulfillment and not as a source of insight and enlightenment.

Under these conditions it is not surprising that besides analytic therapy many alternative forms of treatment for adolescents have been evolved and practiced, such as manipulation of the environment, residential treatment, the setting up of therapeutic communities, etc. Valuable as these experimental approaches are from the practical point of view, they cannot, of course, be expected to contribute to our theoretical insight into the unconscious contents of the adolescent's mind, the structure of his typical disturbances, or into the details of the mental mechanisms by which these latter are maintained.

II. CLINICAL APPLICATIONS

What follows is an attempt to apply at least some of our hard won insights to three of the most pressing problems concerning adolescence.

Is the Adolescent Upset Inevitable?

There is, first, the ever recurrent question whether the adolescent upheaval is welcome and beneficial as such, whether it is necessary and, more than that, inevitable. On this point, psychoanalytic opinion is decisive and unanimous. The people in the child's family and school, who assess his state on the basis of behavior, may deplore the adolescent upset which, to them, spells the loss of valuable qualities, of character stability, and of social adaptability. As analysts, who assess personalities from the structural point of view, we think otherwise. We know that the character structure of a child at the end of the latency period represents the outcome of long drawn-out conflicts between id and ego forces. The inner balance achieved, although characteristic for each individual and precious to him, is preliminary only and precarious. It does not allow for the quantitative increase in drive activity, nor for the changes of drive quality which are both inseparable from puberty. Consequently, it has to be abandoned to allow adult sexuality to be integrated into the individual's personality. The so-called adolescent upheavals are no more than the external indications that such internal adjustments are in progress.

On the other hand, we all know individual children who as late as the ages of fourteen, fifteen or sixteen show no such outer evidence of inner unrest. They remain, as they have been during the latency period, "good" children, wrapped up in their family relationships, considerate sons of their mothers, submissive to their fathers, in accord with the atmosphere, ideas and ideals of their childhood background. Convenient as this may be, it signifies a delay of their normal development and is, as such, a sign to be taken seriously. The first impression conveyed by these cases may be that of a quantitative deficiency of drive endowment, a suspicion which will usually prove unfounded. Analytic exploration reveals that this reluctance to "grow up" is derived not from the id but from the ego and superego aspects of the personality. These are children who have built up excessive defenses against their drive activities and are now crippled by the results, which act as barriers against the normal maturational processes of phase development. They are, perhaps more than any others, in need of therapeutic help to remove the inner restrictions and clear the path for normal development, however, "upsetting" the latter may prove to be.

Is the Adolescent Upset Predictable?

A second question which we are asked to answer frequently concerns the problem whether the manner in which a given child will react in adolescence can be predicted from the characteristics of his early infantile or latency behavior. Apart from the more general affirmative answer given by Ernest Jones (1911), only one among, the authors mentioned above has made clear and positive assertions in this respect. Sigfried Bernfeld (1923), when discussing his protracted type of male adolescence and its characteristics, established the links between this form of puberty and a specific type of infantile development based on the following three conditions: (a) that the frustration of infantile sex wishes has been shattering for the child's narcissism; (b) that the incestuous fixations to the parents have been of exceptional strength and have been maintained throughout the latency period; © that the superego has been established early, has been delineated sharply from the ego, and that the ideals contained in its are invested with narcissistic as well as with object libido.

Other and less precise answers to the same question are scattered through the literature. We find the opinion that, in the majority of cases, the manifestations of the adolescent process are not predictable since they depend almost wholly on quantitative relations, i.e., on the strength and suddenness of drive increase, the corresponding increase in anxiety causing all the rest of the upheaval.

I suggested in another place (1936) that adolescence brings about occasionally something in the nature of a spontaneous cure. This happens in children whose pregenital activities and characteristics remained dominant throughout latency until the increase in genital libido produces a welcome decrease in pregenitality. This latter occurrence, on the other hand, can be matched by a corresponding one which produces the opposite effect: where phallic characteristics have remained dominant during latency, the increase in genital libido produces the effect of an exaggerated and threatening aggressive masculinity. It seems to be generally accepted that a strong fixation to the mother, dating not only from the oedipal but from the preoedipal attachment to her, renders adolescence especially difficult. This latter assertion, on the other hand, has to be correlated with two recent findings of a different nature which we owe to work done in our Hampstead Child Therapy Clinic. One of these findings is derived from the study of orphaned children who were deprived of the relationship of a stable mother figure in the first years. This lack of a mother fixation, far from making adolescence easier, constitute a real danger to the whole inner coherence of the personality during that period. In these cases adolescence is preceded frequently by a frantic search for a mother image; the internal possession and cathexis of such an image seems to be essential for the ensuing normal process of detaching libido from it for transfer to new objects, i.e., to sexual partners.

The second finding mentioned above is derived from the analyses of adolescent twins, in one case children whose twin relationship in infancy had been observed and recorded in minute detail (Burlingham, 1952). In their treatments it transpired that the "adolescent revolt" against the love objects of infancy demands the breaking of the tie to the twin in no lesser degree than the breaking of the tie to the mother. Since this libidinal (narcissistic as well as object-directed) cathexis of the twin is rooted in the same deep layer of the personality as the early attachment to the mother, its withdrawal is accompanied by an equal amount of structural upheaval, emotional upset, and resulting symptom formation. Where, on the other hand, the twin relationship survives the adolescent phase, we expect to see a delay in the onset of maturity or a restrictive hardening of the character of the latency period similar to the instances mentioned above in which the childhood love for the parents withstands the onslaught of the adolescent phase.

To return to the initial question: it seems that we are able to foretell the adolescent reactions in certain specific and typical constellations but certainly not for all the individual variations of infantile personality structure. Our insight into typical developments will increase with the number of adolescents who undergo analysis.

Pathology in Adolescence

This leaves us with a third problem which, to my mind, outweighs the preceding ones so far as clinical and theoretical significance are concerned. I refer to the difficulty in adolescent cases to draw the line between normality and pathology. As described above, adolescence constitutes by definition an interruption of peaceful growth which resembles in appearance a variety of other emotional upsets and structural upheavals.[3] The adolescent manifestations come close to symptom formation of the neurotic or psychotic disorder and merge almost imperceptibly into borderline states, initial, frustrated or fully fledged forms of almost all mental illnesses. Consequently, the differential diagnosis between the adolescent upsets and the true pathology becomes a difficult task.

For the discussion of this diagnostic problem I leave most other authors in the field to speak for themselves and summarize my own impressions based on past and present clinical experience.

In 1936, when I approached the same subject from the aspect of the defenses, I was concerned with the similarity between the adolescent and other emotional disturbances rather than with the differences between them. I described that adolescent upsets take on the appearance of a neurosis if the initial, pathogenic danger situation is located in the superego with neurosis the resulting anxiety being felt as guilt; that they resemble psychotic disturbances if the danger lies in the increased power of the id itself, which threatens the ego in its existence or integrity. Whether such an adolescent individual impresses us, then, as obsessional, phobic, hysterical, ascetic, schizoid, paranoid, suicidal, etc., will depend on the one hand on the quality and quantity of the id contents which beset the ego, on the other hand on the selection of defense mechanisms which the latter employs. Since, in adolescence, impulses from all pregenital phases rise to the surface and defense mechanisms from all levels of crudity or complexity come into use, the pathological results- although identical in structure- are more varied and less stabilized than at other times in life.

Today it seems to me that this structural descripiton needs to be amplified, not in the direction of the similarity of the adolescent to other disorders but in that of their specific nature. There is in their etiology at least one additional element which may be regarded as exclusive to this period and characteristic for it: namely that the danger is felt to be located not only in the id impulses and fantasies but in the very existence of the love objects of the individual's oedipal and preoedipal past. The libidinal cathexis to them has been carried forward from the infantile phases, merely toned down or inhibited in aim during latency. Therefore the reawakened pregenital urges, or-worse still- the newly acquired genital ones, are in danger of making contact with them, lending a new and threatening reality to fantasies which had seemed extinct, but are, in fact, merely under repression.[4] The anxieties which arise on these grounds are directed towards eliminating the infantile objects,i.e., toward breaking the tie with them. Anny Katan (1937) has discussed this type of defense, which aims above all at changing the persons the sense of conflict, under the term of "removal". Such an attempt may succeed or fail, partially or totally. In any case, I agree with Anny Katan that its outcome will be decisive for the success or failure of the other, more familiar line of defensive measures which are directed against the impulses themselves.

A number of illustrations will serve to clarify the meaning of this assumption.

(I) DEFENSE AGAINST THE INFANTILE OBJECT TIES
Defense by displacement of libido.- There are many adolescents who deal with anxiety aroused by attachment to their infantile objects by the simple means of flight. Instead of permitting a process of gradual detachment from the parents to take place, they withdraw their libido from them suddenly and altogether. This leaves them with a passionate longing for partnership which they succeed in transferring to the environment outside the family. Here they adopt varying solutions. Libido may be transferred, more or less unchanged in form, to parent substitutes, provided that these new figures are diametrically opposed in every aspect (personal, social, cultural) to the original ones. Or the attachment may be made to so-called "leaders," usually persons in age between the adolescent's and the parents' generation, who represent ideals. Equally frequent are the passionate new ties to contemporaries, either of the same or of the opposite sex (i.e., homosexual or heterosexual friendships) and the attachments to adolescent groups (or "gangs"). Whichever of these typical solutions is chosen, the result makes the adolescent feel "free," and revel in a new precious sense of independence from the parents who are treated, then, with indifference bordering on callousness.

Although the direction taken by the libido in these instances is, in itself, on lines of normality, the suddenness of the change, the carefully observed contrast in object selection, and the overemphasis on the new

[3]Adolescence of course I snot the only time in life when alterations of physiological nature cause disturbances of mental equilibriu. The same happens in later years in the climacterium; and recently Grete L. Bibring has given a convincing description of similiar damage to the equilibrium of mental forces during pregnancy.

allegiances mark it as defensive. It represents an all too hasty anticipation of normal growth rather than a normal developmental process.

It makes little further difference to the emotional situation whether the libidinal flight is followed by actual flight, i.e., whether the adolescent also "removes" himself bodily from his family. If not, he remains in the home in the attitude of a boarder, usually a very inconsiderate one so far as the older and younger family members are concerned. the other hand, the withdrawal of cathexis from the parents has most decisive consequences for the rest of the defensive processes. Once the infantile objects are stripped of their importance, the pregenital and genital impulses cease to be threatening to the same degree.

Consequently, guilt and anxiety decrease and the ego becomes more tolerant. Formerly repressed sexual; and aggressive wishes rise to the surface and are acted on, the actions being taken outside the family in the wider environment. Whether this acting out will be on harmless, or idealistic, or dissocial, or even criminal lines will depend essentially on the new objects to which the adolescent has attached himself. Usually the ideals of the leader, of the adolescent group, or of the gang, are taken over wholeheartedly and without criticism.

Adolescents of this type may be sent for treatment after their actions have brought them into conflict with their schools, their employers, or the law. As far as psychoanalytic therapy is concerned, they seem to offer little chance for the therapeutic alliance between analyst and patient without which the analytic technique cannot proceed. Any relationship to the analyst and, above all, the transference to him would revive the infantile attachments which have been discarded; therefore the adolescent remains unresponsive. Also, the escape from these attachments has suspended the feeling of internal conflict, at least temporarily; consequently, the adolescent does not feel in need of psychological help. A. Aichhorn had these points in mind when he maintained that adolescents of dissocial and criminal type needed a long period of preparation and inner rearrangement before they could become amenable to analytic treatment. He maintained the latter would be successful only if, during this preparation in a residential setting,

[4]An important clinical instance of this can be found in adolescent girls with anorexia nervosa. Here the infantile fantasies of oral impregnation receive added impetus from the new real possibilities of motherhood opened up by genital development. Consequently, the phobic measures adopted against the intake of food on the one hand and identification with the mother on the other hand are overemphasized to a degree which may lead to starvation.

the adolescent made a new transference of object love, reawakened his infantile attachments, internalized his conflicts once more, in short, became neurotic.

To try an analyze an adolescent in his phase of successful detachment from the past seems to be a venture doomed to failure.

Defense by reversal of affect. A second typical reaction to the same danger situation is, although less conspicuous outwardly, more ominous in nature inwardly.

Instead of displacing libido from the parents- or more likely, after failing to do so- the adolescent ego may defend itself by turning the emotions felt toward them into their opposites. This changes love into hate, dependence into revolt, respect and admiration into contempt and derision. On the basis of such reversal of affect the adolescent imagines himself to be "free" but, unluckily for his peace of mind and sense of conflict, this conviction does not reach further than the conscious surface layer of his mind. For all deeper intents and purposes he remains as securely tied to the parental figures as he had been before; acting out remains within the family; and any alterations achieved by the defense turn out to his disadvantage. There are no positive pleasures to be derived from the reversed relationships, only suffering, felt as well as inflicted. There is no room for independence of action, or of growth; compulsive opposition to the parents proves as crippling in this respect as compulsive obedience to them can prove to be.[5] Since anxiety and guilt remain undiminished, constant reinforcement of defense is necessary. This is provided in the first place by two methods: denial (of positive feeling) and reaction formations (churlish, unsympathetic, contemptuous attitudes). The behavioral picture that emerges at this stage is that of an uncooperative and hostile adolescent.

Further pathological developments of this state of affairs are worth watching. The hostility and aggressiveness, which serve as a defense against object love in the beginning, soon become intolerable to the ego, are felt as threats, and are warded off in their own right. This may happen by means of projection; in that case the aggression is ascribed to the parents who, consequently, become the adolescent's main oppressors and persecutors. In the clinical picture this appears first as the adolescent's suspiciousness and, when the projections increase, as paranoid behavior.

Conversely, the full hostility and aggression may be turned away from the objects and employed inwardly against the self. In these cases, the adolescent's display intense depression, tendencies of self-abasement and self-injury, and develop or even carry out, suicidal wishes.

During all stages of this process, personal suffering is great and the desire to be helped intense. This, in itself, is no guarantee that the adolescent in question will submit to analytic therapy. He will certainly not do so if treatment is urged and initiated by the parents. Whenever this happens, he will consider analysis as their tool, extend his hostility or his suspicions to include the person of the analysts, and refuse cooperation. The chances are better if the adolescent himself decides to seek help and turns to analysis, as it were, in opposition to the parents' wishes. Even so, the alliance with the analyst may not be of long duration. As soon as a true transference develops and the positive infantile fantasies come into consciousness, the same reversal of affect tends to be repeated in the analytic setting. Rather than relive the whole turmoil of feelings with the analyst, many adolescent patients run away. They escape from their positive feelings, although it appears to the analyst that they break off treatment in an overwhelmingly strong negative transference.

Defense by withdrawal of libido to the self.-To proceed in the direction of increasing pathology:

Withdrawal of libido from the parents, as it has been described above, does not, in itself, decide about its further use, or fate. If anxieties and inhibitions block the way toward new objects outside the family, the libido remains within the self. There, it may be employed to cathect the ego and superego, thereby inflating them. Clinically this means that ideas of grandeur will appear, fantasies of unlimited power over other human beings, or major achievement and championship in one or more fields. Or, the suffering and persecuted ego of the adolescent may assume Christ-like proportions with corresponding fantasies of saving the world.

On the other hand, the cathexis may become attached to the adolescent's body only and give rise there to the hypochondriacal sensations and feelings of body changes that are well known clinically from initial stages of psychotic illness.

In either case analytic therapy is indicated as well as urgent. Treatment will dispel the appearance of severe abnormality if it reopens a path for the libido, either to flow backwards and recathect the original infantile objects, or to flow forward, in the direction described above, to cathect less frightening substitutes in the environment.

What taxes the analyst's technical skill in these cases is the

---

ˢS.Ferenczi has pointed to this effect of "complusive disobedience" many years ago.

withdrawn state of the patient, i.e., the problem of establishing an initial relationship and transference. Once this is accomplished, the return from narcissistic withdrawal to object cathexis will relieve the patient, at least temporarily. I believe, there are many cases where the analyst would be wise to be content with this partial success without urging further treatment. A further, and deeper, involvement in the transference may well arouse all the anxieties described above and, again, lead to abrupt termination of the analysis due to the adolescent's flight reaction.

Defense by regression - The greater the anxiety aroused by the object ties, the more elementary and primitive is the defense activity employed by the adolescent ego to escape them. Thus, at the extreme height of anxiety, the relations with the object world may be reduced to the emotional state known as "primary identification" with the objects. This solution with which we are familiar from psychotic illnesses implies regressive changes in all parts of the personality, i.e., in the ego organization as well as in the libido. The ego boundaries [6] are widened to embrace parts of the object together with the self. This creates in the adolescent surprising changes of qualities, attitudes and even outward appearance. His allegiance to persons outside himself betrays itself in these alterations of his own personality (i.e., his identifications) rather than in an outflow of libido. Projections, together with these identifications, dominate the scene and create a give-and-take between the self and object which has repercussions on important ego functions. For example, the distinction between the external and internal world (i.e., reality testing) becomes temporarily negligible, a lapse in ego functioning which manifests itself in the clinical picture as a state of confusion.

Regression of this kind may bring transitory relief to the ego by emptying the oedipal (and many of the preoedipal) fantasies of their libidinal cathexis.[7] But this lessening of anxiety will not be longlived. Another and deeper anxiety will soon take its place which I have characterized on a former occasion (1951) as the fear of emotional surrender, with the accompanying fear of loss of identity.

(II) DEFENSE AGAINST IMPULSES

Where the defenses against the oedipal and preoedipal object ties fail to achieve their aim, clinical pictures emerge which come nearest to the borderline toward psychotic illness. *The "ascetic" adolescent.*- One of

---

[6] See P. Federn (1952) and, following him T. Freeman et al. (1958).

these the "ascetic" adolescent, I have described before as fighting all his impulses, preoedipal and oedipal, sexual and aggressive, extending the defense even to the fulfillment of the physiological needs for food, sleep, and body comfort. This, to me, seems the characteristic reaction of an ego, driven by the blind fear of overwhelming id quantities, an anxiety which leaves no room for the finer distinctions between vital or merely pleasant satisfactions, the healthy or the morbid, the morally permitted or forbidden pleasures. Total war is waged against the pursuit of pleasure as such. Accordingly, most of the normal processes of instinct and need satisfaction are interfered with and become paralyzed. According to clinical observation, adolescent asceticism is, with luck, a transitory phenomenon. For the analytic observer it provides precious proof of the power of defense, i.e., of the extent to which the normal, healthy drive derivatives are open to crippling interference by the ego.

On the whole, analytic treatment of the ascetic type does not present as many technical difficulties as one would expect. Perhaps, in these individuals, defense against the impulses is so massive, that they can permit themselves some object relationship to the analyst and thus, enter into transference.

The "uncompromising" adolescent.-Another, equally abnormal adolescent, is described best as the "uncompromising" type. The term, in this instance, does refer to more than the well-known conscious, ideas, refuse to make concessions to the more practical and reality-adapted attitudes of their elders, and take pride in their moral or aesthetic unrelenting position adopted by many young people who stand up for their principles. "Compromise," with these adolescents, includes processes which are as essential for life as, for example, the cooperation between impulses, the blending of opposite strivings, the mitigation of id strivings by interference from the sode of the ego. One adolescent whom I observed in analysis did his utmost, impursuit of this impossible aim, to preven any interference of his mind with his body, of his activity with his passivity, his loves with his hates, his realities with his fantasies, the external demands with his internal ones, in short, of his ego with his id.

In treatment this defense was represented as a strong resistance against any "cure," the idea of which he despised in spite of intense suffering. He understood correctly that mental health is based in the last resort on harmony, i.e., on the very compromise formations which he was trying to avoid.

III. THE CONCEPT OF NORMALITY IN ADOLESCENCE

Where adolescence is concerned, it seems easier to describe its pathological manifestations than the normal processes. Nevertheless, there are in the above exposition at least two pronouncements which may prove useful for the concept: (1) that adolescence is by its nature an interruption of peaceful growth, and (2) that the upholding of a steady equilibrium during the adolescent process is in itself abnormal. Once we accept for adolescence disharmony within the psychic structure as our basic fact, understanding becomes easier. We begin to see the upsetting battles which are raging between id and ego as beneficent attempts to restore peace and impulses, or against the object cathexis, begin to appear legitimate and harmony. The defensive methods which are employed either against the normal. If they produce pathological results, this happens not because of any malignancy in their nature, but because they are overused, overstressed, or used in isolation. Actually, each of the abnormal types of adolescent development, as it is described above, represents also a potentially useful way of regaining mental stability, normal if combined with other defenses, and if used in moderation.

To explain this last statement in greater detail: I take it that it is normal for an adolescent to behave for a considerable length of time in an inconsistent and unpredictable manner; to fight his impulses and to accept them; to ward them off successfully and to be overrun by them; to love his parents and to hate them; to revolt against them and to be dependent on them; to be deeply ashamed to acknowledge his mother before others and, unexpectedly, to desire heart-to-heart talks with her; to thrive on imitation of and identification with others while searching unceasingly for his own identity to be more idealistic, artistic, generous, and unselfish than he will ever be again, but also the opposite: self-centered, egoistic, calculating. Such fluctuations between extreme opposites would be deemed highly abnormal at any other time of life. At this time they may signify no more than that an adult structure of personality takes a long time to emerge, that the ego of the individual in question does not cease to experiment and is in no hurry to close down on possibilities. If the temporary solutions seem abnormal to the onlooker, they are less so, nevertheless, than the hasty decisions made in other cases for one-sided suppression, or revolt, or flight, or withdrawal, or regression, or asceticism, which are responsible for the truly pathological

[7]See in this connection M. Katan (1950).

developments described above.

While an adolescent remains inconsistent and unpredictable in his behavior, he may suffer, but he does not seem to me to be in need of treatment. I think that he should be given time and scope to work own solution. Rather, it may be his parents who need help and guidance so as to be able to bear with him. There are few situations in life which are more difficult to cope with than an adolescent son or daughter during the attempt to liberate themselves.

IV. SUMMARY

In the foregoing paper the author has reviewed and summarized some of the basic literature on adolescence, as well as her own views on the subject. Her former description of the defensive processes in adolescence has been amplified to include specific defensive activities directed against the oedipal and preoedipal object ties.

BIBLIOGRAPHY

Adatto, C. P. (1938), Ego Reintegration Observed in Analysis of Late Adolescents. *Int.J.Psa.*, XXXIX.

Aichhorn,A. (1925), *Wayward Youth*. New York: Viking Press, 1918.

Balint,M. (1934), Der Onanieabgewohnungskampf in der Pubertat. *Ztsch. psa.Pad.*,VIII.

Bernfeld,S. (1923), Uber eine typische Form der mannlichen Pubertat. *Imago*, IX. (1924), *Vom dichterischen Schaffen der Jugend*. Wien: Internationaler Psychoanalytischer Verlag.

(1935), Uber die einfache mannliche Pubertat. *Ztsch. psa. Pad.*, IX.

(1938), Types of Adolescence. *Psa. Quart.*, VII.

Bornstein, B.(1949), Discussion following the presentation of Phyllis Greenacre's paper (see Greenacre, 1950) at the New York Psychoanalytic Society. Abstracted in *Psa.Quart.*, XVIII, p 277.

Burlingham,D. (1952), *Twins*. New York: International Universities Press.

Buxbaum,E. (1933), Angstausserungen von Schulmadcen im Pubertatsalter. *Ztsch. psa Pad.*, VIII.

(1915), Transference and Group Formation in Children and Adolescents. *Psychoanalytic Study of the Child*, I.

Deutsch,H. (1941), *The Psychology of Women*, 1. New York: Grune &

Stratton.
Eissler, K. R. (1950), Ego-Psychological Implications of the Psychoanalytic Treatment of Delinquents. *Psychoanalytic Study of the Child*, V.
   (1953), Notes upon the Emotionality of a Schizophrenic Patient and Its Relation to problems of technique. *Psychoanalytic Study of the Child*, VIII.
Erikson, E. H.(1946), Ego Development and Historical Change. *Psychoanalytic Study of the Child*, II.
Federn, P. (1912), Contribution in: *Die Onanie. 14 Beitrage zu e i n e r Diskussion der Weiner Psychanalytischen Vereinigung.* Wiesbaden: J. F. Bergmann.
   (1952), *Ego Psychology and the Psychoses.* New York: Basic Books.
Fenichel, O. (1938), Review of The Ego and the Mechanisms of Defence. *Int. J. Psa.* XIX.
   (1945), *The Psychoanalytic Theory of Neurosis.* New York: Norton.
Ferenczi, S. (1912), Contribution in: *Die Onanie. 14 Beitrage zu einer Diskussion der Wiener Psychoanalytischen Vereinigung.* Wiesbaden: J. F. Bergmann.
Fraiberg, S. (1955), Some Considerations in the Introduction to Therapy in Puberty. *Psychoanalytic Study of the Child.*, X.
Freeman, T., Cameron, L. J.& McGhie, A. (1958), *Chronic Schizophrenia.* New York: International Universities Press.
Freud, A. (1927), *Psycho-Analytical Treatment of Children.* London: Imago Publishing Co., 1946.
   (1936), *The Ego and the Mechanisms of Defense.* New York: International Universities Press,1946. See Chapters X and XI.
   (1951), A Connection between the States of Negativism and of Emotional Surrender (*Horigkeit*), Paper read at the International Psycho-Analytical Congress, Amsterdam, August 1951. Summary in *Int. J. Psa.*, XXXIII, 1952, p. 265.
Freud, S. (1905), Three Essays on the Theory of Sexuality. *Standard Edition*, VII. London: Hogarth Press, 1953.
   (1912), Contribution in: *Die Onanie. 14 Beitrage zu einer Diskussion der Weiner Psychoanalytischen Vereinigung.* Weisbaden: J. F. Bergmann.
Friedlander, K. (1941), Uber Kinderbucher und ihre Funktion in Latenz und Vorpubertat. *Int. Ztsch. Psa. S Imago*, XXVI.

Geleerd, E. R. (1957), Some Aspects of Psychoanalytic Technique in Adolescents. *Psychoanalytic Study of the Child*, Xll.

Gitelson, M. (1948), Character Synthesis: The Psychotherapeutic Problem in Adolescence. Am. J. Orthopsychiat., XVIII.

Greenacre, P. (1950), The Prepuberty Trauma in Girls. *Psa. Quart.*, XIX.

Harnik, J. (1923), The Various Developments Undergone by Narcissism in Men and Women. *Int. J. Psa.*, V, 1924.

Hartmann, H., Kris, E., & Loewenslein, R. M. (1946), Comments on the Formation of Psychic Structure. *Psychoanalytic Study of the Child*, II.

Hoffer, W. (1946), Diaries of Adolescent Schizophrenics. *Psychoanalytic Study of the Child* , II.

Jones, E. (1922), Some Problems of Adolescence. *Papers on Psycho-Analysis*. London:Bailliere, Tindall & Cox, fifth edition, 1948.

Katan-Angel, A. (1937), The Role of Displacement in Agoraphobia. *Int. J. Psa.* XXXII,   1951.

Katan, M. (1950), Structural Aspects of a Case of Schizophrenia. *Psychoanalytic Study of the Child*, V.

Klein, M. (1946), *The Psycho- Analysis of Children*. London: Hogarth Press.

Kris, E. (1938), Review of The Ego and the Mechanisms of Defence. *Int. J. Psa.*, XIX

Lampl-de Groot, J. (1950), On Masturbation and Its Influence on General Development. *Psychoanalytic Study of the Child*, V.

Landauer, R. (1935), Die Ichorganisation in der Pubertat. *Ztsch. psa. Pad.*, IX.

Lander, J. (1942), The Pubertal Struggle Against the Instincts. *Am. J. Orthopsychiat.*, XII.

Maenchen, A. (1916), A Case of Superego Disintegration. *Psychoanalytic Study of the Child*, II.

Noshpitz, J. (1957), Opening Phase in the Psychotherapy of Adolescents with Character Disorders. *Bull. Menninger Clin.*, XXI.

Reich, A. (1950), On the Termination of Analysis. *Int. J. Psa.*, XXXI.

Root, N. N. (1957), A Neurosis in Adolescence. *Psychoanalytic Study of the Child*, XII.

Schmideberg,M. (1931), Psychoanalytisches zur Menstruation. *Ztsch. psa. Pad.*, V.

Spiegel, L. A. (1951), A Review of Contributions to a Psychoanalytic Theory of Adolescence. *Psychoanalytic Study of the Child* , VI.

Wittels, F. (1949), The Ego of the Adolescent. In: *Searchlights on*

Delinquency, ed. K. R. Eissler. New York: International Universities Press.

CHAPTER THREE
CHARACTER FORMATION IN ADOLESCENCE

Peter Blos

The problem of character formation is of such a vast scope that almost any aspect of psychoanalytic theory is related to it. This fact tells us at the outset that we deal with a concept of enormous complexity or with integrative processes of the highest order. It is a sobering and welcome limitation to concentrate on the adolescent period and investigate, in this circumscribed domain, whether this particular stage of development affords us insight into the formative process of character, and consequently throws light on the concept of character in general. It would not be the first time in the history of psychoanalysis that the nature of a psychic phenomenon becomes illuminated by the study of its formation.

Whoever has studied adolescence, regardless of theoretical background, has been aware of changes in the maturing personality that are generally identified with character formation. Even the untutored observer of youth, or the adult who retrospectively contemplates his own adolescence, cannot fail to notice that, with the termination of adolescence, a new mode of dealing with the exigencies of life is in evidence. Behavior, attitudes, interests, and relationships appear more predictable, show a relatively greater stability, and tend to become irreversible, even under stress.

The psychoanalytic observer of adolescence can attest to these findings. However, he asks himself which psychic mechanisms or which maturational processes are at work in character formation. The process of formation, indeed, raises the question of "what takes form" and "what gives form"; furthermore, what are the preconditions for the formation of character, and why and to what extent does it occur at the stage of adolescence? Precursors of character can be discerned abundantly in childhood. However, we not attribute to these rather habitual ways in which the ego deals with id, superego and reality the designation of character, because the integrated, rather fixed pattern of its disparate components is still lacking. Due to the adolescent forward step in the organization of character traits, Gitelson (1948) referred to "character synthesis: as the essential therapeutic task

Presented at the Fall Meeting of the American Psychoanalytic Association, New York, December 16, 1967.

during the adolescent period. Empirically, we all have come to similar conclusions. However, I believe that the formation of character in adolescence is the outcome of psychic restructuring or, in other words, it is the manifest sign of a completed, not necessarily complete, passage through adolescence. We all had occasion to observe how the analysis of an adolescent, especially of the older adolescent, moves toward its termination by the silent emergence of character. What do we mean by this obvious something that emerges? This question forces us to consider some pertinent aspects of psychoanalytic characterology.

Character Traits and Character

The etymological root of the word "character" in the Greek verb of "to furrow and to engrave" has always remained part of the concept of character in regard to the permanency and fixity of patterns of design. These permanencies are represented, in terms of personality, by distinctive traits or qualities and by typical or idiosyncratic ways of conducting oneself. Even the style of life and temperamental attitudes were here and there brought into the broad scope of character.

In the psychoanalytic literature on character we encounter an imprecise and inconsistent use of terms. The interchangeable use of "character," "character type," and "character trait" has been particularly confusing. We can, roughly, distinguish four approaches to classical psychoanalytic characterology. In one approach (Freud, 1908; Abraham, 1921, 1924, 1925; Jones, 1918; Glover, 1924), the character trait is traced to a specific level of drive development or drive fixation (e.g., oral character traits); in another (W. Reich, 1928,1930), the defensive aspect of the ego represents the decisive factor (e.g., the reactive character); in the third (Freud, 1939), it is the fate of object libido that determines the character (e.g., the narcissistic or anaclitic character); and in the fourth (Erikson, 1946), it is the influence of environment, culture, and history that engraves a patterned and preferential style of life on people (the psychosocial definition of character). Of course, these four determinants of character traits and of character are not mutually exclusive; on the contrary, they appear in various admixtures and combinations. The salient feature of each characterological formation is the implicit ego syntonicity and absence of conflict, as distinct from neurotic symptom formation, and the patterned fixity of the characterological organization.

Two widely accepted definitions of character read as follows: "... typical mode of reaction of the ego towards the id and the outer world" (Reich, 1929, p.149).
"... the habitual mode of bringing into harmony the tasks presented by internal demands and by the external world, is necessarily a function of... the ego" (Fenichel, 1945,p. 467).

Character originates in conflict, but, by its very nature, it prevents the arousal of signal anxiety through the codification of conflict solutions. The automatization of dealing with idiosyncratic danger situations represents a considerable forward step in personality integration and functioning. Indeed, character formation can be conceptualized from an adaptive point of view, and clinical evidence in support of such a thesis is easily obtainable. The economic gain inherent in character formation frees psychic energy for the expansion of adaptive inventiveness and the actualization of human potentialities. The economic gain involved in character formation was stated clearly by Freud (1913): "repression either does not come into action [in character formation] or smoothly achieves its aim of replacing the repressed by reaction-formations and sublimations" (p. 323). Having observed these substitutions in the analysis of adolescents, I wonder whether the counter cathexis of the reactive (defensive) character does restrict rather than expand the adaptive scope of self- realization. I shall return to this question.

The transformation of drive fixations into character traits is so universal and so well documented that it requires little comment. It might, however, not be superfluous to mention that instinctual predilections in combination with special sensitivities constitute inherent aspects of human development. When drive fixations are transformed into character traits, the qualitative and quantitative factors due to endowment bestow on each character a highly individualistic countenance.

We are familiar with the host of character traits that take their origin, separately or mixed, in the various levels of psychosexual development. Secondarily, the ego makes use of such proclivities by drawing them into its own realm and employing them for its own purposes. We then speak of the sublimation type of character, If the instinctual predilection gives rise to conflict, then the automatization of defenses marks the character in some decisive fashion, as is exemplified in the reactive character. We can see that the fixed ego attitude of dealing with danger (e.g., "avoidances") has a broader, more inclusive scope than a character trait derived from drive transformations (e.g., "obstinacy"). Yet, we cannot discern such circumscribed, enduring, and fixed ego reactions in children because the child's ego remains partly and significantly interlocked with parental and environmental object dependencies up to the age of puberty . We certainly can discern distinct character traits in the child. However, what appears as character in childhood is mainly a pattern of ego attitudes, stabilized by identifications, which we know, can undergo a most radical revision during adolescence. Here lies one further reason for the fact that character formation and adolescence are synonymous. precocious character consolidation occurring before puberty should be looked at as abnormal development, because it precludes that essential elasticity and flexibility of psychic structure without which the adolescent process can not take its normal course.

The distinction between character traits and character corresponds with the developmental line of demarcation drawn by adolescence. Character traits, then are not identical character, per se, nor is character simply the sum total of character traits. Of course, we can trace in each individual oral, anal, urethral, and phallic- genital characteristics or character traits, but neither one of these characteristics suffices, neither can it do justice to a person's character as a monolithic structure. If we recognize in a person a degree of orderliness, stubbornness, and frugality, we no doubt are confronted with anal character traits. However, we hesitate to call that person an anal character unless we know more about the economic, structural, and dynamic factors, indeed the degree to which these traits are still cathected with a anal erotism and the extent to which these traits became emancipated from infantile bondage and in time acquired functions far removed from their genetic source.

We are reminded here of Hartmann's (1952) statement that defensive ego functions can lose their defensive nature in time and become valuable and integral ego assets serving a far wider function than the original defensive one. Similarly, it can be said that "reactive character formation, originating in defense against the drives, may gradually take over a host of other functions in the framework of the ego" (Hartmann, 1952, p. 25), namely, remain a part of the personality despite the fact that its original *raison d'etre* has vanished. Hartmann's point of view opens up two avenues of thought: either the defensive nature of the character trait is altered because it is emptied of its counter cathexis; or, on the other hand, the id component is afforded a nonconflictual gratification in the exercise and maintenance of character. Could it be that the attainment of the genital level of drive maturation facilitates either one of these outcomes? Furthermore, could it be assumed that these transitions or modifications of character traits into character formation are the cardinal achievement of adolescence? We certainly ascertain in character formation integrative processes, structurings and patternings that belong to a different order than a mere bundling together of traits, attitudes, habits and idiosyncrasies. Lampl-de-Groot (1963), following a similar line of thought, modified the earlier definitions of character (W. Reich. 1929; Fenichel, 1945) by saying that character is the habitual way in which integration is achieved.

The Function of Character

My remarks, up to this point, about character formation have carried an implicit assumption that should now be stated directly and affirmatively. It should, however, be borne in mind that these propositions are laid down here only in order to pave the road to the central theme of this investigation, namely, the relationship between the adolescent process and character formation.

It is assumed that character, as a definitive component of adult psychic structure, performs an essential function in the mature psychic organism. This function is manifested in the maintenance of psychosomatic homeostasis, in patterned self-esteem regulation (A.Reich, 1958), in the stabilization of ego identity (Erikson, 1956) and in the automatization of threshold and barrier levels, both shifting in accordance with the intensity of internal or external stimuli. This regulatory function includes the containment of affective fluctuations within a tolerable range, including depression, as a major determinant in character formation (Zetzel, 1964).

The more complex a psychic formation, the more elusive to the observer becomes the total configuration or organization. The concept of character is a case in point. We have to content ourselves with the study of components or, more precisely, with a description of the whole in terms of the function of its constituent parts. The whole can be assembled as a psychic entity from such fractional comprehension (Lichtenstein, 1965). Two investigative approaches are now open to us; one, to study observable functions in order to impute structure (dynamic, economic principle); and, two, to trace the growth of a psychic formation and see how it comes into its own (genetic principle). These approaches are not the result of an arbitrary choice, but they are forced upon us by the nature of our subject. Character formation is, generally speaking, an integrative process and as such aims at the elimination of conflict and anxiety arousal. We are reminded of Anna Freud's (1936) statement that the ego cannot be studied when it is in harmony with id, superego, and the outer world; it reveals its nature only when disharmony between the psychic institutions prevails. We are faced with a similar dilemma in studying character. Here, too, we can clearly describe pathological character formation, while the typical process of character formation remains elusive. In the analysis of adolescents we cannot fail to notice how character takes shape silently, how it consolidates proportions of the severance from and dissolution of infantile ties: like Phoenix rising from its ashes.

Let us return now to the question why the formation of character occurs at the stage of adolescence or, rather, at the termination of adolescence. Generally we recognize developmental progression by the appearance of new psychic formations as he consequence of differentiating processes. Drive and ego maturation always leads to a new and more complex personality organization. Adolescent drive progression to the adult genital level presupposes a hierarchical arrangement of the drives, as is reflected in the formation of forepleasure. Ego maturation, distinctly influenced but not wholly determined by drive progression, is reflected in qualitative cognitive advances as described by Inhelder and Piaget (1958). looking at the development and maturation in terms of differentiating and integrative processes, we can now ask the question which of these processes in adolescence are preconditional for character formation.

I shall approach this problem by investigating some aspects of typical adolescent drive and ego progression that make character formation not only possible but mandatory for the stabilization of the newly attained personality organization of adulthood. If it is possible to describe character in terms of observable functions, and character formation in terms preconditions or of epigenetic sequences or abandoned developmental stages, then the aim of this exploration would be closer in our reach. Zetel (1964) has emphasized the developmental aspect of character formation and speaks of a developmental task, which, I think, belongs to the phase of late adolescence. Zetel's expansion of the definition of character formation is noteworthy; she stated: "Character formation ... includes the whole range of solutions, adaptive or maladaptive, to recognized developmental changes" (p.153).

The Adolescent Process and Character Formation

I have chosen four adolescent developmental changes which I have chosen to be closely related to character formation. In fact, character formation remains stunted or takes on some abnormal slant if these challenges are not met with reasonable competence. It should be evident that I look at character formation from a developmental point of view and see in it a normative formation that reflects the result of progressive ego and drive development at adolescence. One might compare it of the emergence of the latency period as a result of the oedipal resolution.

Whenever the oedipal stage is prolonged beyond its proper timing, latency development remains incomplete or defective. We are accustomed to consider the decline of the oedipus complex as a precondition for latency to come into its own. In a comparable and similar perspective I introduce here four developmental preconditions without which adolescent character formation cannot take its course.

The Second Individuation

The first precondition which I shall discuss encompasses what has been called the loosening of the infantile object ties (A. Freud, (1958), a process which in its wider scope, I have conceptualized as the second individuation process of adolescence (Blos, 1967). The developmental task of this process lies in the disengagement of libidinal and aggressive cathexes from the internalized infantile love and hate objects. We know how closely infantile object relations are interwoven with psychic structure formation as demonstrated, for example, by the transformation of object love into identification. I do not have to remind you that object relations activate and form ego nuclei around which subsequent experiences coalesce, and that they induce and sharpen idiosyncratic sensitizations, inclusive of preferences and avoidances. The most dramatic and fateful formation derived from object relations is, of course, the superego. Conflicts of the infantile period and of childhood give rise to many character traits and attitudes which can, at times, be easily observed *in status nascendi.*

We recognize in the disengagement from infantile object ties the psychological counterpart to the attainment of somatic maturity, brought about by the biological process of puberty. The psychic formations that not only were derived from object relations, but more or less, still maintain close instinctual ties to infantile object representations are affected, often catastrophically, by the second individuation of adolescence. Again, the superego demonstrates, by the degree of its disorganization or disintegration at adolescence, the affective affinity of this structure to infantile object ties. I can only hint here at the fact that many controls and adaptational function pass over from the superego to the ego ideal, namely, to a narcissistic formation. The love of the infant's parent is, partially at least, replaced by the love of the self or its potential perfection.

The psychic restructuring, implicit in what I have described above, cannot be accomplished without regression. The relentless striving toward increasing autonomy through regression forces us to view this kind of regression in adolescence as regression in the service of development, rather than in the service of defense. In fact, adolescent analysis demonstrates convincingly not only the adolescent's defense against phase-specific regression, but also the task of the analysis to facilitate regression.

Adolescent regression not only is unavoidable, it is obligatory, namely phase specific. Adolescent regression in the service of development brings the more advanced ego of the adolescent into contact with infantile drive positions, with old conflictual constellations and their solutions with early object relations and narcissistic formations. We might say that the personality functioning which was adequate for the child undergoes a selective overhaul. The ego's advanced resourcefulness is brought to bear on this task.

In the course of adolescent psychic restructuring the ego draws drive propensities and superego influences into its own realm, integrating these disparate elements into an adaptive pattern. The process of the second individuation proceeds via regressive recathexis of pregenital and preoedipal positions. They are, so to say, revisited, lived through again, but with the difference that the adolescent ego, being in a vastly more mature state vis-a-vis infantile drives and conflicts is able to bring about shifts in the balance between ego and id. New identifications ("the friend," "the group," etc.) take over super-ego functions, episodically or lastingly. The adolescent's emotional and physical withdrawal from, or opposition to, his world of childhood dependencies and security measures makes him, for some time, seek a protective cover in passionate, but usually transient, peer associations. We then observe shifting identifications with imitative and restitutive connotations as expressed in posture, gait, gesture, attire, speech, opinion, value system, etc. Their shifting and experimental nature is a sign that character has not yet been formed, but it also indicates that social adaptation has transcended the confines of the family, its milieu and tradition. These social way stations, significant as they are, have outlasted their usefulness with the unfolding and implementation of a life plan, with the capacity for adult object relations, and with a realistic projection of the self into the future. Then we know that a consolidation of the personality has come about, that a new forward step in internalization has been taken, that inner consistencies and uniformities have become stabilized, that behavior and attitudes have acquired an almost predictable countenance, reliance, and harmony.

Residual Trauma

I shall now turn to the second precondition for adolescent character which will throw light on the function of character. I hope to show that the character takes over homeostatic functions from other regulatory agencies of childhood.[1] In this connection we have to consider the effect of trauma on adolescent character formation. The usage of the term "trauma" in this paper corresponds with Greenacre's (1967) definition. She writes: "In my own work I have not limited my conception of trauma to sexual (genital) traumatic events, or circumscribed episodes, but have included *traumatic conditions* i.e. *any conditions which seem definitely unfavorable, noxious, or drastically injurious to the development of the young individual"* (128).

Clinical observation gave rise to the theoretical formulations that follow. The analysis of older adolescents has demonstrated to me that the resolution of the neurotic conflict, the weaning from infantile fantasies, will bring the analytic work to a good end, without, however, having eliminated all residues of the pathogenetic foundation on which the illness rested. These residues remain recognizable in special sensitivities to certain stimuli, external or internal, as well in affinities to, or avoidances of, experiences and fantasies, or in somatic proclivities, despite the fact that all these aspects were dealt with exhaustively in analysis. By the end of the analysis, these residues have lost their noxious valence due to ego and drive maturation. in spite of this, they do not require constant containment, which is to say, they still are factors to be reckoned with in the maintenance of psychic homeostasis. it is my contention that the automatization of this containment process is identical with the function of, or more precisely, with a part function of character. Such sensitizations to special danger situations of a

---

[1] Again, I have to condense here what I developed elsewhere (1962, pp. 132-140).

permanent traumatic valence are to be found, for example, in object loss, passive dependency, loss of control, decline of self- esteem, and other structurally and affectively injurious conditions.

It is assumed here that trauma is a universal human condition during infancy and early childhood, leaving, under the most favorable circumstances, a permanent residue. The adolescent process, unable to overcome the disequilibrizing effect of this residue, assimilates it through characterological stabilization, namely by rendering it ego syntonic. I draw here on Freud's distinction between a positive and a negative effect of trauma, a reaction that leads to the reactive character formation via avoidances, phobias, compulsions and inhibitions. The positive effects "are attempts to bring the trauma into operation once again- that is, to remember the forgotten experience, ... to make it real, to experience a repetition of it... [The effects] may be taken up in into what passes as a normal ego and, as permanent trends in it, may lend it unalterable character traits" (Freud, 1939, p. 75).

The high noon of this integrative achievement lies in the terminal period of adolescence when the enormous instability of psychic and somatic functions gradually gives way to an organized and integrated mode of operation. The residual trauma cease to alert the ego repetitiously via signal anxiety once it has become an integral part of the ego. Their residual trauma has become an organizer in the process of character formation. A state of helplessness and vigilance has become counteracted by character formation. Character, then, is identical with patterned responses to signal anxiety or, generally, with the conquest of residual trauma; not with its disappearance, nor its avoidance, but with its continuance within an adaptive formation.

Residual trauma lends its persistent and relentless push toward actualization to that formation within the personality which we designate as character. Due to its origin character always contains a compulsive quality; it lies beyond choice and contemplation, is self- evident and compelling: "Here I stand, I cannot do otherwise' (Luther). the psychic energy required for character to take form is derived I part, from the cathexis which the residual trauma contains. Those adolescents who sidestep the transformation of residual trauma into character formation project the danger situation into the outside world and thus avoid the internal confrontation with it. By failing to internalize the danger situation, the chance for coming to terms with it is fortified. this impasse results in what Erikson (1956) has described as the adolescent moratorium, which leads either to belated character formation or to a pathological outcome. We gain the impression that the formation of character encompasses more than superego influences, identifications or defenses. We are now ready to state that in character formation there is an integrative principle at work which bends the various contributing and confluent components to a broadening of the ego's secondary autonomy. Erikson's concept of ego identity (1956) belongs in this realm of clinical impressions.

In the analysis of older adolescents we can observe the luxuriant fantasy life of adolescence shriveling up with the consolidation of character. Greenacre (1967) comments on the fact that whenever a traumatic experience was associated with an underlying fantasy, the fixation on the trauma is more persistent than in cases where the trauma was bland and incidental. Is it possible that in adolescent character formation not only the experiential side of the residual trauma, but also the fantasy associated with it, are absorbed in the ego organization? The thought has often been expressed that instinctual drives find expression in the exercise of a so-called healthy character. At any rate, we are now willing to say that the characterological stabilization of residual trauma advances the independence of man from his environment, from which the traumatic injury originally emanated at a time when pain was identical with the outside of the self or with the nonself.

Ego Continuity

I now come to he third precondition for adolescent character formation. Again, clinical observation has shown the direction and cleared the path to a conceptual formulation. I have described certain cases of adolescent acting out in which the maladaptive behavior represents an effort via action language to contradict a distortion of the family history that was coercively forced upon the child's mind. I have designated such conditions as "family myth" (1963). it differs from the classical family romance in that the distortion is forced on the child from the outside, calling in question the validity of the child's own perception, The study of a considerable number of such cases has convinced me that adolescent development can be carried forward only if the adolescent ego succeeds in establishing a historical continuity within its realm. If this is prevented, a partial foreclosure of adolescent development follows, namely, the psychic restructuring of adolescence remains-incomplete. Besides delinquency, much of the quandary and adventurousness of youth as well as its creativity, especially literary, productions can be studied from this point of view.

The establishment of historical ego continuity appears, of course, in any analysis, but in adolescent analysis it has an integrative and growth-stimulating effect that lies beyond conflict resolution. One adolescent spoke for many in saying that one cannot have a future without having a past. Again, we observe a tendency toward internalization or, conversely, toward a disengagement (on the ego level) from the adult caretaking environment (usually the family) which has acted as the trustee and guardian of the immature ego of the child. It seems that ego maturation, along the lines I have just described gives rise to the subjective sense of wholeness and inviolability during the adolescent years, when the envelope of the family has outlived its usefulness. Of course, the sense of wholeness and inviolability has much in common with the psychological qualities that we ascribe to the reflection of character on subjective feeling states.

Sexual Identity

In order to complete the set of preconditions that promote adolescent character formation, a fourth one has to be mentioned, namely, the emergence of sexual identity. While gender identity is established at an early age, it has been my contention that sexual identity with definitive, i.e., irreversible, boundaries appears only belatedly as the collateral of sexual maturation at puberty. Before physical sexual maturity is attained, the boundaries of sexual identity remain fluid. Indeed, a shifting or ambiguous sexual identity, within limits, is the rule rather than the exception. This is more apparent in the girl than in the boy. I have only to remind you of the acceptability, socially and personally, of the tomboy stage in the girl and of the deep repression of breast envy in the preadolescent boy. At any rate, puberty represents the demarcation line beyond which bisexual admixtures to gender identity become incompatible with progressive development. Clinically, this can easily be observed in the adolescent's growing capacity for heterosexual object finding and in the decline of masturbation, both of which advance parallel with the with formation of sexual identity.

It is not the purpose of this paper to trace the origin or the resolution of bisexuality. But it needs to be said that, as long as the ambiguity or, indeed, the ambivalence of sexual identification lasts , the ego cannot escape being affected by the ambiguity of the drives. The maturational exigencies of puberty which normally lead to integrative processes of increasing complexity are not able to perform their function as long as sexual ambiguity prevails; that is to say, maturational processes will be defeated all along the line. Subjectively, this is experienced by the adolescent as identity crisis or identity diffusion, using Erikson's (1956) terms. In the pursuit of our subject we would conclude that the formation of character presupposes that sexual identity formation has advanced along a narrowing path, leading to masculinity or femininity.

At this juncture, in late adolescence and postadolescence, we can observe how persistently remnants of the bisexual orientation have been debarred from genital expression and been absorbed in character formation. The role of the ego ideal, the heir of the negative oedipus complex (Blos, 1963), so important and decisive at this turning point of late adolescence, can only be hinted at because the pursuit of it, relevant as it might be, exceeds the limits of this exposition.

The Genealogy of Character

The four preconditions which I have outlined rest on antecedents that reach back into the earliest history of individual life. We have good reason to assume that, beyond these experiential aspects, that are embedded in the character structure components that hark back to biological givens. It follows from this view that adolescent character formation is affected, adversely or beneficially, by constitutional conditions as well as by infantile antecedents and their lifelong effect on psychic structure and conflict. The characterological stabilization of drive and ego vicissitudes is not, however, identical with character. The four, by no means definitive preconditions must be transcended in some fashion before the homeostatic function of this new formation that we can call character is regulated. The credentials of character are to be found in the postadolescent developmental level which, if attained, renders character formation possible; in other words, character formation reflects the structural accommodations which have brought the adolescent process to a close. The extent to which the four preconditions have been fulfilled, or the extent to which the four developmental challenges have been met, will determine the autonomous or defensive nature of the character that ensues. With the termination of childhood during the pubertal period, adult somatic of structure and functioning are reached; this attainment has its psychological counterpart in the consolidation of the personality or in the formation of character.

It must have become clear during this presentation that in talking about character, one is constantly tempted to speak of healthy or pathological character formation. I have not offered in my schema any explicit accommodation of the so-called character disturbances, character disorders. or the vast spectrum of the pathological character. Proceedings from clinical observation of adolescents and on the basis of analytic data, I have arrived at conclusions and formulations which I have submitted. These have to be brought into harmony with observations of similar substance but derived from other characterological phenomena and other periods of life. This lies beyond the scope of my investigation.

The Evolutionary Aspect of Character

I realize with apprehension that I have not heeded my initial admonition too well and have burdened this presentation with a vast array of theoretical concerns. This is the risk one runs in discussing character formation. There remains, however, still one further comment on this subject to which I shall now turn.

I have approached character formation as a corollary to drive and ego maturation at the stage of puberty. In doing so I have lifted it out of its ontogenetic matrix and assigned to it a function that is commensurate with the concurrent biological, namely sexual, maturation and the morphological attainment of adult status. Each stage of maturation increases the complexity of the psychic organization. Character reflects on the level of personality development the attainment of the highest form of physical structure formation and functioning. References, explicit or implicit, to the complex structure and function of character can be found in the analytic literature that attributes to character a holistic, integrative principle of various designations: the synthesizing function of the ego, fitting together (Hartmann), identity formation, organizing principle, consolidation process, the self, the whole person, etc. All these connotations have in common the subjective experience that one's character is identical with one's self. Psychic life cannot be conceived without it, just as physical life is inconceivable without one's body. One feels at home in one's character, or *mutatis mutandis* one's character is one's home and is, indeed, a dependable and reliable protector of the self. One accepts a shortcoming of one's character the way one accepts a physical imperfection. One does not like it, but there it is. When Lawrence Durrell was asked whether he is aware of any specific weakness as a writer, he gave the following answer: "My great weaknesses come from my character, not from lack of talent; I am hasty, rash; impulsive at moments when I should be timid, reserved and objective, and vice versa. My prose and poetry clearly show this weakness". (*Realities,*

April, 1961). We cannot fail to detect in this statement a note of pride for possessing the courage to accept one's weakness. A comment by Lichtenstein (1965) is pertinent to this observation: "Insofar as we are perceiving such an invariant as a characteristic of our own inner world (Hartmann), we tend to refer to it as the *experience* (Erlebnis) of our Self" (p. 119). Character formation establishes new invariants in the psychic life, and thus heightens and stabilizes the experience of the self. This, essentially identical, experience was derived in childhood from the invariants -reliability and sameness-of the environment.

Character structure renders the psychic organism less vulnerable than it had ever been before, and the maintenance of this structure is secured against any interference from any quarter, internal or external. If must be, one dies for it before letting it die. The overvaluation of one's own character makes it apparent that character is cathected with narcissistic libido and that narcissistic gratification is a legitimate gain derived from the exercise of character.

I am aware that I have spoken above in anthropomorphic metaphor instead of psychological concepts. This I shall correct by pointing out that the four preconditions are essentially a forward step in internalization and consequently in a furtherance of independence from the environment. A higher level of integration is thereby reached which contains new homeostatic possibilities. In this sense, we can say, applying the genetic point of view, that the utter dependence of the human infant on environmental, protective stability has achieved in character formation its contra position, namely, the internalization of a stable, protective environment. While content and pattern of character are socially determined, it is only internalization that renders the psychic organism greatly independent from those forces that brought it into existence. While character structure is of a most durable and irreversible kind, only a degree of openness and flexibility assures its enrichment and modulation during adult life.

The evolutionary aspect of character formation lies in the internalization of dependencies and the formation of a progressively complex psychic structure. The function of character lies in the maintenance of this psychic structure that is self- regulatory, namely, automatized, and thus reduces the infliction of psychic injury to a minimum. It goes without saying that the level of psychic organization thus achieved facilitates the unfolding of man's boundless potentialities.

In character formation we observe, on the ontogenic level of personality development, an evolutionary principle that has its parallel. On the phylogenetic level, in advancing independence of the organism from the conditions of its environment. This evolution has reached its apex in man. Claude Bernard (1859) has expressed this principle by saying that "The constancy of the internal environment is the condition of the free life". In this sense, we can view character formation in an evolutionary perspective and contemplate it as a closed system that, through its operation, maintains its adaptive function, which is to facilitate the creative use of the human potentiality. The process of internalization and automatization in character formation establish and stabilize the psychic mileau, thus enabling man to shape his environment, singly and collectively, by impressing on it those conditions that correspond most favorably with the inviolability and integrity of his personality.

Bibliography

Abraham, K. (1921), Contributions to the Theory of the Anal Character. In: *Selected Papers on Psycho-Analysis*. London: Hogarth Press, 1927, pp. 370-392.
- (1924), The Influence of Oral Erotism on Character-Formation. In: *Selected Papers on Psycho-Analysis*. London: Hogarth Press, 1927, pp. 893-406.
- (1925), Character-Formation on the Genital Level of Libido. In: *Selected Papers on Psycho-Analysis*. London: Hogarth Press, 1927, pp. 407-417.
Blos, P. (1962), *On Adolescence: A Psychoanalytic Interpretation*. New York: Free Press of Glencoe.
- (1963), The Concept of Acting Out in Relation to the Adolescent Process. *J. Amer. Acad. Child Psychiat.*, 2:118-136.
(1967), The Second Individuation Process of Adolescence. *Psychoanal. Study of the Child*, 22:162-188.
Erikson, E. H. (1946), Ego Development and Historical Change. *Psychoanal. Study of the Child*, 2:359-396.
-(1956), The Problem of Ego Identity. *J. Amer. Psa. Assn.*, 4:56-121.
Fenichel, O. (1945), *The Psychoanalytic Theory of Neurosis*. New York: Norton.
Freud, A. (1936), *The Ego and the Mechanisms of Defense*. New York: International Universities Press, rev. ed., 1966.
(1958), Adolescence. *Psychoanal. Study of the Child*, 13:255-278.

Freud, S. (1908), Character and Anal Erotism. *Standard Edition*, 9:167-175. London: Hogarth Press, 1959.

-(1913), The Disposition to Obsessional Neurosis. *Standard Edition*, 12: 311-396. London: Hogarth Press, 1958.

-(1931), Libidinal Types. *Standard Edition*, 21:215-220. London: Hogarth Press, 1961.

-(1939), Moses and Monotheism. *Standard Edition*, 23:3-137. London: Hogarth Press, 1964.

Gitelson, M. (1948), Character Synthesis: The Psychotherapeutic Problem of Adolescence, *Amer. J. Orthopsychiat.*, 18:422-431.

Glover, E. (1924), Notes on Oral Character Formation. In: *On the Early Development of Mind.* New York: International Universities Press, 1956, pp. 25-46.

Greenacre, P. (1967), The Influence of Infantile Trauma on Genetic Patterns. In:*Psychic Trauma*, ed. S. S. First. New York: Basic Books, pp. 108-153.

Hartmann, H. (1952), The Mutual Influences in the Development of Ego and Id. *Psychoanal. Study of the Child*, 7:9 30.

Inhelder, B. & Piaget, J. (1958), *The Growth of Logical Thinking.* New York: Basic Books.

Jones, E. (1918), Anal-Erotic Character Traits. In: *Papers on Psychoanalysis.* Baltimore: Williams & Wilkins, 5th ed., 1948, pp. 413 437.

Lampl-de Croot, J. (1963), Symptom Formation and Character Formation. *Int. J. Psa.*, 44:1-11.

Lichtenstein, H. (1965), Towards a Metapsychological Definition of the Concept of Self. *Int. J. Psa.*, 46:117-128.

Reich, A. (1958), A Character Formation Representing the Integration of Unusual Conflict Solutions into the Ego Structure. *Psychanal. Study of the Child,*, 13:309-323.~

Reich, W. (1928), On Character Analysis. In: *The Psychoanalytic Reader*, ed. R. Fliess. New York: International Universities Press, 1948, pp. 129-147.

-(1929), The Genital Character and the Neurotic Character. In: *The Psychoanalytic Reader*, ed. R. Fliess. New York: International Universities Press, 1948, pp. 148-169.

        -(1930), Character Formation and the Phobias of Childhood. In: *The Psychoanalytic Reader*, ed. R. Fliess New York: International Universities Press, 1948, pp.170-182.

Zetzel, E. R. (1964), Symptom Formation and Character Formation. *Int. J. Psa.*, 45:151-154.

CHAPTER FOUR
ADOLESCENCE
STRUGGLING THROUGH THE
DOLDRUMS

Donald Winnicott

There is at this present time a world-wide interest in adolescence and the problems of the adolescent. In almost all countries there are adolescent groups that make themselves evident in some way or other. Many studies of this phase of development are being made, and there has arisen a new literature, either of autobiography written by the young, or of novels that deal with the lives of teenage boys and girls. It is safe to assume that there is a connection between this development in our social awareness and the special social conditions of the times we live in. One thing that must be recognized at the start by those who explore in this area of psychology is the fact that the adolescent boy or girl does not want to be understood. Adults must hide among themselves what they come to understand of adolescence. It would be absurd to write a book for adolescents on adolescence because this period of life is one which must be lived, and it is essentially a time of personal discovery. Each individual is engaged in a living experience, a problem of existing.

Cure for Adolescence

There exists one real cure for adolescence, and only one, and this cannot be of interest to the boy or girl who is in the throes. The cure for adolescence belongs to the passage of time and to the gradual maturation processes; these together do in the end result in the emergence of the adult person. This process cannot be hurried or slowed up, though indeed it can be broken into and destroyed, or it can wither up from within, in psychiatric illness.

We do sometimes need to remind ourselves that although adolescence is something that we have always with us, each adolescent boy or girl grows up in the course of a few years into an adult. Parents know this better than some sociologists do, and public irritation with the phenomenon of adolescence can easily be evoked by cheap journalism and by the public pronouncements of persons in key positions, with adolescence referred to as a problem, and the fact that each individual adolescent is in process of becoming a responsible society-minded adult left out of the argument.

THEORETICAL STATEMENT

There is a considerable measure of agreement among those concerned with dynamic psychology with regard to a general statement of adolescence in terms of the emotional development of the individual.

The boy or girl in this age-phase is dealing with his or her personal puberty changes. He or she comes to the developments in sexual capacity and to secondary sexual manifestations with a personal past history, and this includes a personal pattern in the organization of defenses against anxiety of various kinds. In particular, *in health*, there has been in each individual an experience before the latency period of a full-blooded Oedipus complex, that is to say, of the two main positions in the triangular relationship with the two parents (or parent substitutes); and there have been (in the experience of each adolescent) organized ways of warding off distress or of accepting and tolerating the conflicts inherent in these essentially complex conditions.

Also derived from the experiences of each adolescent's early infancy and childhood are certain inherited and acquired personal characteristics and tendencies, fixations to pregenital types of instinctual experience, residues of infantile dependence and of infantile ruthlessness; and further, there are all manner of illness patterns associated with failures of maturation at Oedipal and preOedipal levels. Thus the boy or girl comes up to puberty with all patterns predetermined, because of infantile and early childhood experiences, and there is much that is unconscious, and much that is unknown because it has not yet been experienced.

There is room for a great deal of variation in individual cases as to the degree and type of the problem that may result, but the general problem is the same: How shall this ego organization meet the new id advance? How shall the pubertal changes be accommodated in the personality pattern that is specific to the boy or girl in question? How shall the adolescent boy or girl deal with the new power to destroy and even to kill, a power which did not complicate feelings of hatred at the toddler age? It is like putting new wine into old bottles.

The Environment

The part played by the environment is immensely significant at this stage, so much so that it is best, in a descriptive account, to assume the continued existence and interest of the child's own father and mother and of wider family organizations. Many of the difficulties of adolescents for which professional help is sought derive from environmental failure, and this fact only emphasizes the vital importance of the environment and of the family setting in the case of the vast majority of adolescents who do in fact achieve adult maturity, even if in the process they give their parents headaches.

Defiance and Dependence

A characteristic of the age group under examination is the rapid alternation between defiant independence and regressive dependence, even a coexistence of the two extremes at one moment of time.

The Isolation of the Individual

The adolescent is essentially an isolate. It is from a position of isolation that a beginning is made which may result in relationships between individuals, and eventually in socialization. In this respect the adolescent is repeating an essential phase of infancy, for the infant is an isolate, at least until he or she has repudiated the not-me, and has become set up as a separated-off individual, one that can form relationships with objects that are external to the self and outside the area of omnipotent control. It could be said that before the pleasure-pain principle has given way to the reality principle the child is isolated by the subjective nature of his or her environment.

Young adolescents are collections of isolates, attempting by various means to form an aggregate through the adoption of an identity of tastes. They can become grouped if they are attacked as a group, but this is a paranoid organization reactive to the attack; after the persecution the individuals return to their state of being an aggregate of isolates.

Sex Prior to Readiness for Sex

The sex experiences of younger adolescents are colored by this phenomenon of isolation; and also by the fact that the boy or girl does not yet know whether he or she will be homosexual, heterosexual, or simply narcissistic. In many cases there is a long period of uncertainty as to whether a sex urge will turn up at all. Urgent masturbatory activity may be at this stage a repeated getting rid of sex, rather than a form of sex experience, and indeed compulsive heterosexual or homosexual activities may themselves at this age serve the purpose of a getting rid of sex or a discharge of tensions, rather than of a form of union between whole human beings. Union between whole human beings is more likely to appear, first, in aim-inhibited sex play, or in affectionate behavior with the accent on sentiment. Here again is the personal pattern, waiting to join up with the instincts, but in the long meanwhile there has to be found some form of relief from sexual tension; and compulsive masturbation would be expected in a high proportion of cases, if we had an opportunity to know the facts. (A good motto for any investigator of the subject would be this: whoever asks questions must expect to be told lies.)

It is certainly possible to study the adolescent in terms of the ego coping with id changes, and the practicing psycho-analyst must be prepared to meet this central theme, either manifest in the child's life or displayed cautiously in the material presented by the child in the analytic setting, or in the child's conscious and unconscious fantasy and in the deepest parts of the personal psychic or inner reality. Here, however, I will not pursue this approach, because my purpose is to survey adolescence in another way and to attempt to relate today's urgency of the adolescent theme to the social changes that belong to the past fifty years.

THE TIME FOR ADOLESCENCE

Is it not a sign of the health of a society that its teenagers are able to be adolescent at the right time, that is to say, at the age that covers pubertal growth? Among primitive peoples either the pubertal changes are hidden under taboos or else the adolescent is turned into an adult in the space of a few weeks or months by certain rites and ordeals. In our present society, adults are being formed by natural processes out of adolescents who move forward because of growth tendencies. This may easily mean that the new adults of today have strength and stability and maturity.

Naturally, there must be a price to pay for this. The many adolescent breakdowns call for toleration and treatment; and also this new development puts a strain on society, for it is distressing for adults who have themselves been defrauded of adolescence to watch the boys and girls in a state of florid adolescence all round them.

THREE SOCIAL CHANGES

In my opinion there are three main social developments that have altered the whole climate for adolescents in adolescence:

(I) *Venereal disease* is no longer a bogy. The spirochaete and the gonococcus are no longer (as they were certainly felt to be fifty years ago) agents of a punishing God. Now they can be dealt with by penicillin and by appropriate antibiotics.[1]

(ii) *The development of contraceptive techniques* has given the adolescent the freedom to explore. This freedom is very new, the freedom to find out about sexuality and sensuality when there is not only an absence of a wish for parenthood, but also, as there nearly always is, a wish to avoid bringing into the world an unwanted and unparented baby. Of course, accidents happen and will happen, and these accidents lead to unfortunate and dangerous abortions or to the birth of illegitimate children. But in examining the problem of adolescence we must accept the fact, I suggest, that the modern adolescent can explore, if he or she has a mind to, the whole area of sensuous living, without suffering the mental agony that accidental conception involves. This is only partly true because the mental agony associated with the fear of an accident remains, but the problem has been altered in the course of the last thirty years by this new factor. The mental agony now, we can see, comes from the individual child's innate guilt sense. I do not that every child has an innate guilt sense, but I mean that, in health, the child develops in a very complicated way a sense of right and wrong, a sense of guilt, and ideals, and an idea of what he or she wants for the future.

(iii) *The atom bomb* is perhaps producing even more profound changes than the two characteristics of our age that I have listed so far. The atom bomb affects the relationship between adult society and the adolescent tide, which seems to be for ever coming in. We have to carry on now on the basis that there *is not going to be another war*. Now it can be argued that there might be a war at any minute in some place in the world, but we know that we can no longer solve a social problem by organizing for a new war. So there is no longer any basis on which we can justify the provision of strong military or naval discipline for our children, however convenient it might be for us to be able to do so.

Here comes the effect of the atom bomb. If it no longer makes sense to deal with our difficult adolescents by preparing them to fight for their King and Country, then that is another reason why we are thrown back on the problem that there is this adolescence, a thing in itself. So now we have got to 'dig' adolescence.

The adolescent is pre-potent. In the imaginative life the potency of man is not just a matter of the active and passive of intercourse. It includes a man's victory over a man and a girl's admiration of the victor. All this now, I am suggesting, has to be wrapped up in the mystique of the cafe bar and in the occasional disturbance with knives. Adolescence has to contain itself much more than it has ever had to do before, and itself is pretty violent material - rather like the repressed unconscious of the individual, not so beautiful if opened out to the world.

When we think of the notorious atrocities of modern youth, we must weigh against them all the deaths that belong to the war that is not, and that is not going to be; against all the cruelty that belongs to the war that is not going to be; and against all the free sexuality that belongs to every war that has ever been but is not going to be again. So adolescence is here with us, which is evident, and it has come to stay.

These three changes are having an effect on our social concern, and this shows clearly in the way in which adolescence comes into prominence as something that is no longer to be hustled off the stage by false maneuvers, like conscription.

THE UNACCEPTABILITY OF THE FALSE SOLUTION

It is a prime characteristic of adolescents that they do not accept false solutions. This fierce morality on the basis of the real and the false belongs also to infancy and to illness of schizophrenic type.

The cure for adolescence is the passage of time, a fact which has very little meaning for the adolescent. The adolescent looks for a cure that is immediate, but at the same time rejects one 'cure' after another because some false element in it is detected.

Once the adolescent can tolerate compromise, he or she may discover various ways in which the relentlessness of essential truths can be softened. For instance, there is a solution through identification with parent figures; or there can be a premature maturity in terms of sex; or there can be a shift of emphasis from sex to physical prowess in athletics, or from the bodily functions to intellectual attainment or achievement. In general, adolescents reject these helps, and instead they have to go through a sort of *doldrums area*, a phase, in which they feel futile and in which they have not yet found themselves. We have to watch this happening. But a total avoidance of these compromises, especially of the use of identifications and vicarious experience, means that each individual must start from scratch, ignoring all that has been worked out in the past history of our culture.

Adolescents can be seen struggling to start again as if they had nothing they could take over from anyone. They can be seen to be forming groups on the basis of minor uniformities, and on the basis of some sort of group adherence which belongs to locality and to age. Young people can be seen searching for a form of identification which does not let them down in their struggle, *the struggle to feel real*, the struggle to establish a personal identity, not to fit into an assigned role, but to go through whatever has to be gone through. They do not know what they are going to become. They do not know where they are, and they are waiting. Because everything is in abeyance, they feel unreal, and this leads them to do certain things which feel real to them, and which are only too real in the sense that society is affected.

We do in fact get very much caught up with this curious thing about adolescents, *the mixture of defiance and dependence*. Those looking after adolescents will find themselves puzzled as to how boys and girls can be defiant to a degree and at the same time so dependent as to be childish, even infantile, showing patterns of the infantile dependence that dates from their earliest times. Moreover, parents find themselves paying out money to enable their children to be defiant against themselves. This is a good example of the way in which those who theorize and write and talk are operating in a layer that is different from the layer in which adolescents live, and in which parents or parent-substitutes are faced with urgent problems of management. The real thing here is not the theory but the impact of the one on the other, the adolescent and the parent.

ADOLESCENT NEEDS

So it is possible to gather together the needs that adolescents manifest:

The need to avoid the false solution.
The need to feel real or to tolerate not feeling at all.
The need to defy in a setting in which dependence is met and can be relied on to be met.
The need to prod society repeatedly so that society's antagonism is made manifest, and can be met with antagonism.

HEALTHY ADOLESCENCE AND ILLNESS PATTERNS

That which shows in the normal adolescent is related to that which shows in various kinds of ill person. For example:

1. The need to avoid the false solution corresponds with the psychotic patient's inability to compromise; compare also psychoneurotic ambivalence, and the deceptiveness and self-deception of health.
2. The need to feel real or not to feel at all is related to psychotic depression with depersonalization.
3. The need to defy corresponds with the antisocial tendency as it appears in delinquency.

From this it follows that in a group of adolescents the various tendencies tend to be represented by the more ill members of the group. For example, one member of a group takes an overdose of a drug, another lies in bed in a depression, another is free with the flick- knife. In each case the aggregate of isolates is grouped behind the ill individual, whose extreme symptom has impinged on society. Yet, for the majority of the individuals who are involved there is not enough drive behind the tendency to bring the symptom into inconvenient existence and to produce a social reaction.

The Doldrums

To repeat: if the adolescent is to get through this development stage by natural process, then there must be expected a phenomenon which could be called *adolescent doldrums*. Society needs to include this as a permanent feature and to tolerate it, to react actively to it, in fact to come to meet it, *but not to cure it*. The question is, has our society the health to do this?

Complicating this issue is the fact that some individuals are too ill (with psychoneurosis or depression or schizophrenia) to reach a stage of emotional development that could be called adolescence, or they can reach it only in a highly distorted way. I have not included in this account a description of severe psychiatric illness as it appears at this age level; nevertheless, one type of illness cannot be set aside in any statement about adolescence, namely, delinquency.

Adolescence and the Antisocial Tendency

It is revealing to study the close relationship that exists between the normal difficulties of adolescence and the abnormality that may be called the antisocial tendency. The difference between these two states lies not so much in the clinical picture that each presents as in the dynamic, in the aetiology, of each. At the root of the antisocial tendency there is always a deprivation. It may simply be that the mother, at a critical time, was in a withdrawn state or depressed, or it may be that the family broke up. Even a minor deprivation, if it occurs at a difficult moment, may have a lasting result because it over strains the available defenses. Behind the antisocial tendency there is always some health and then an interruption, after which things were never the same again. The antisocial child is searching in some way or other, violently or gently, to get the world to acknowledge its debt; or is trying to make the world re-form the framework which got broken up. At the root, therefore, of the antisocial tendency there is this deprivation. At the root of adolescence in general it is not possible to say that there is inherently a deprivation, and yet there is something which is the same, but, being less in degree and diffused, it just avoids over straining the available defenses. So that the group that the adolescent finds to identify with, or in the aggregate of isolates that forms into a group in relation to a persecution, the extreme members of the group are acting for the total group. All sorts of things in the adolescents' struggle - the stealing, the knives, the breaking out and the breaking in, and everything - all these have to be contained in the dynamic of this group, sitting round listening to jazz, or having a bottle party. And, if *nothing happens*, the individual members begin to feel unsure of the reality of their protest, and yet they are not in themselves disturbed enough to do the antisocial act which would make things right. But if in the group there is an antisocial member, or two or three, willing to do the antisocial thing which produces a social reaction, this makes all the others cohere, makes them feel real, and temporarily structures the group. Each individual member will be loyal and will support the one who will act for the group, although not one of them would have approved of the thing that the extreme antisocial character did.

I think that this principle applies to the use of other kinds of illness. The suicidal attempt of one of the members is very important to all the others. Or one of the group cannot get up; he is paralyzed with depression, and has got a record-player playing very doleful music; he locks himself in his room and nobody can get near. The others all know that this is happening, and every now and again he comes out and they have a bottle party or something, and this may go on all night or for two or three days. Such happenings belong to the whole group, and the group is shifting and the individuals are changing their groups; but somehow the individual members of the group use the extremes to help themselves to *feel real*, in their struggle to get through this doldrums period.

It is all a problem of *how to be adolescent during adolescence*. This is an extremely brave thing for anybody to be, and some of these people are trying to achieve it. It does not mean that we grown-ups have to be saying: 'Look at these dear little adolescents having their adolescence; we must put up with everything and let our windows get broker.' that is not the point. The point is that we are challenged, and we meet the challenge as part of the function of adult living. But we meet the challenge rather than set out to cure what is essentially healthy.

The big challenge from the adolescent is to the bit of ourselves that has not really had its adolescence. This bit of ourselves makes us resent these people being able to have their phase of the doldrums, and makes us *want to find a solution for them*. There are hundreds of false solutions. Anything we say or do is wrong. We give support and we are wrong, we withdraw support and that is wrong too. We dare not be 'understanding'. But in the course of time we find that this adolescent boy and this adolescent girl have come out of the doldrums phase and are now able to begin identifying with society, with parents, and with all sorts of wider groups, without feeling threatened with personal extinction.

1 I remember clearly a conversation with a girl, sometime after the first world war. She told me that it was only the fear of venereal disease that had kept her from being a prostitute. She was horrified at the idea I put forward in a simple conversation that venereal disease might one day be preventable or curable. She said that she could not imagine how she could have got through her adolescence (and she was only just coming through it) without this fear, which she had used in order to keep straight. She is now the mother of a large family and would be called a normal sort of person; but she had to come through her adolescent struggle and the challenge of her own instincts. She had a difficult time. She did a bit of thieving and lying, but she came through. But she held on to the venereal disease deterrent.

CHAPTER FIVE
YOUTH IN TURMOIL:
AN INTERPERSONAL PERSPECTIVE

Edwin Kasin

I would feel more secure if I were going to present this evening a single case report. I could then tell you with reasonable certainty that he said this and I said that, he did this and I did that, and after a few months or years we had come to some agreement as to what was bothering him about living and why. But I have chosen a much larger field for discussion, namely, "Youth in Turmoil," which general as it may be, I am confident gives you a fairly clear idea as to the phenomenon I wish to discuss.

Quite recently, although gradually developing over a somewhat longer period, great restlessness and malaise have come over our young population, a demoralization and dissatisfaction that have assumed epidemic proportions. Newspapers, books, periodicals, learned journals have been filled with an ever-increasing number of articles and studies of these young people behaving in strange and disturbing ways. They are described as alienated, disaffected, rebellious, rejecting, self-absorbed, in a moral crisis, in a crisis of faith, and so on. They are lauded as the finest generation of young people we have ever raised, and they are equally referred to as effete intellectual snobs.

I have read a great deal of the reportage and theorizing on these developments and, what is more, encountered these phenomena in healthy, bright, intelligent, eager young people-the children of friends and associates moving into the period of youth-as well as all around me in the streets and public places, and in referrals to my practice, which made me wonder what I knew that would justify the supposition that I was an expert in the field. Thirty years ago we might have labeled them schizophrenics, or psychopaths, or borderlines, and tried to mold them back into some shape of "normality" while wondering what their "terrible" parents had foisted upon them in the way of mental pathology.

In the last ten years there have appeared broad phenomena known as juvenile delinquency, the beat scene, the hippie scene, the activist scene, revolt on the campus, the drug scene, dropping out et cetera, events that on the whole constitute and reflect a tragic waste of good human potential. I

Presented at the William Alanson White Institute, New York City, on March 11, 1970.

have wondered if there was a nuclear meaning to all these phenomena Could I identify the problem, for the slight peace of mind such activity would give me? Eldridge Cleaver's statement in *Soul on Ice*, "If you're not part of the solution, you're part of the problem" seemed a distillation of interpersonal wisdom. Tonight's presentation is my very modest attempt to be part of the solution, to which I bring my interest in the developmental method of understanding events in human.

In Sullivan's thinking there were two main goals in living: (1) Fulfillment of biological needs, which he called the pursuit of satisfactions; and (2) avoidance of social disapproval (or anxiety), which he called the pursuit of security. Thus, the personal history of any individual would include the history of progressive maturation of needs in an interpersonal matrix in a society that facilitated or thwarted such development, and the patterning effects on the individual of such interaction. As a result certain experiences (facilitated) are more or less in awareness, and others, which encountered serious disapproval, remain out of awareness or, as we say, become dissociated.

In tracing from its beginnings the story of the growing individual's interaction with his enlarging world, I am going to focus on some of the vicissitudes which, in my mind, throw some clarity on the current scene.

Let us first consider the infant. At the beginning the needs of the infant are fairly simple. To breathe, to be warm, to be fed, and to be free of pain. Now, it would be very impressive if I were to confront you at this moment with a live infant deprived of any one of these necessities, or failing that, a movie depicting the same. My words, especially since I am talking about theory, may easily move you toward somnolence; but a live howling infant, or a reasonable facsimile of one would be very impressive indeed. It would convey more than the statement that the needs are simple, but they are pressing and urgent. This urgency is best demonstrated in connection with the need for oxygen. The low storage of this substance makes its absence most dramatically felt; if deprived of it the infant would be in gravest danger to life.

Any threat to the survival of bodily integrity carries with it a felt aspect, fear (Sullivan's definition), which can move rapidly to terror. Not so obvious to most of us, the satisfaction of the other needs are just as urgent. It certainly is obvious to the explorer in the desert or the Arctic, the native of Biafra, or the soldier in combat. Because of fortunate location (possibly temporary) in time and place, most of us are spared the experience of the urgency of starvation, freezing, or pain, although mutilation seems to be becoming an increasing possibility even in the best urban areas.

I am trying here to convey the urgency of needs. Currently there is a great interest in the subject of aggression. I might say a great deal of this discussion of aggression impresses me as confused and confusing. Curiously enough, you will find scarcely a mention of this term in Sullivan's later works, and I think he was fairly thorough and utterly observant. I believe that in some way the curiosity will inevitably turn to the subject of need-urgency. In other words, the problem is not how to deal with aggression as a force in man, but how to deal with the urgency of need fulfillment. When and if this has been done, I suspect all that will remain to be said about aggression will be considered under the rubric of mastery.

In infancy then, anoxia, leading to fear, then terror, calls out earlier survival mechanisms: vigorous muscular activity accompanied by rage reactions, ultimately leading to convulsions and discharges of the autonomic system as the organism utilizes motivational patterns possibly useful in an earlier organization of the central nervous system for survival purposes. Deprivation of the other needs would lead in this direction except for a particular dynamism that has been built in, as it were, that is, the dynamism of apathy, in which needs suddenly attenuate and the infant falls into a sort of sleep. To paraphrase Sullivan's dramatic example (1953, p. 56), a hungry baby kicks and shrieks and, as his needs mount his rage increases; then apathy, a curious safety device, operates and the needs are attenuated. To the extent that there is a felt aspect to apathy, I suppose it is depression. But I qualify this because, if you are really apathetic, you feel very little; only as you emerge somewhat from apathy do you feel depression. I mention this because it has relevance later on; we see less hysteria (Freud), obsessionalism, perhaps even schizophrenia, but increasing depression in our practices.

I am getting a little ahead of the story when I tell you I have just described an infant in turmoil. Long before social pressures on the infant become significant, we may see these aspects of unsatisfied need, namely, fear, rage and apathy. Ultimately the mothering one arrives, the needs are met, peace once more returns, and growth continues. Fortunately for the infant, there is a mothering one. And in discussing these early experiences of infancy Sullivan formulates what he calls the theorem of tenderness (1953, pp 39-40), stating in effect that the infant communicates his needs (or the tension of need) by crying; this crying communicates to the mother that the infant has needs, which she experiences as the tension of the need to give tenderness. Lo, the infant takes care of his mother's need by being satisfied, so they both have given and taken. That is the interpersonal bond with which life in this world begins.

If we return for a moment to that infant in turmoil: There will shortly appear the first prehension or dimly perceived experience of what later will be identified as the fear of abandonment. Each of us is perpetually in thrall to this fear, avoiding it only to the extent that we have well rationalized, well practiced techniques for being amongst our fellows. It is the other side, if you will, of our need for contact with significant others. In a childhood when social isolation is taught to all children (go up to your room and so forth), it is a powerful tool for enforcing necessities; and in the juvenile period, when the need for compeers matures, social isolation can become a veritable nightmare. Thus the need to belong, to be where others can meet one's needs, is a powerful and perjuring fact of life.

What I have been discussing is the absent- mother or the absent- other phenomenon, the urgency of needs in the period of life before what Sullivan called the quiet miracle of preadolescence. Thus far I have said little about anxiety except to indicate its connection with social disapproval. It is hardly likely that a mother who is exposed to the infant's turmoil will not feel she has failed in her social responsibility as a mother; this is equivalent to her being anxious. In this fashion she induces anxiety in the infant, and considerably complicates his life. But note that he was already well into his tumultuous pattern simply on the basis of his unfulfilled need. She may, at least theoretically, be utterly indifferent, in which case he perishes, or she may view him as the embodiment of evil, a monster sent to plague her, which at this utterly dependent period all hut spells his doom.

As we move on to the next stage, development assumes broader dimensions. The infant has learned language and is beginning to learn to talk. Now the mothering ones feel it their responsibility to raise the child to be a member of society. They are going to train him to live in their world. From now on he will have to bend the knee somewhat, or suffer social disapproval, called anxiety. He will be hampered in his free exploration and in working out direct expression of his needs, if and when these conflict with his society. The undoing of the aberrations of adaptations in this period have constituted the main and more successful work of psychiatrists in the relatively recent past, and probably will for some time to come. But successful psychiatry now seems to be in some jeopardy of becoming irrelevant to a large segment of the so-called youth in turmoil.

I want to go back at this juncture to a brief discussion of Sullivan's understanding of the stages of development. He identified six stages: infancy, childhood, juvenile, pre-adolescence, adolescence (early and late), and adulthood. Each succeeding period is initiated by the maturation within the individual of a new biological need. Thus, when the infant picks up the rudiments of language, signaling his readiness for training, childhood begins. Some years later a need for companionship with others his own age will develop. So pressing is this need that in the event of social isolation the juvenile will invent fantasy companions. In this stage too, there will develop the skills of social accommodation, competition, and cooperation, including the introduction and comparison of one's own and the other's ways of life, carried over from childhood. Then comes the stage of preadolescence when the isophilic need for intimacy matures, followed by adolescence and the puberty change in which the capacity to integrate lustful integrations occurs; onward to a patterning of the sexual relationship with a person of the opposite sex. Finally adulthood or fully mature living arrives.

I have just given only a brief statement about the significant need which matures and primarily characterizes each developmental period. It is important to understand that each stage is predestined, if you will, by biological imperatives. Thus, since the beginning of human history, or perhaps human living in primitive tribes, in ancient times, Egyptian culture, ancient Indian culture, and so on through the Greek and Roman eras, feudal times and the Renaissance and of course up to and including modern societies. In each and every society of man, it is foredained that these periods of development will occur and manifest themselves as behavior in the interest of the fulfillment of needs.

What will vary from culture to culture is the freedom with which one can explore and rationally understand activities connected with the satisfaction of these needs, and their ramifications. Each culture has a body of unreasoned dogma (or religion) and a body of so-called priests or elders who, set the limits on what one can be free about investigating. Tendencies that one could not indulge freely would most often be provided for in the religion, so that some sublimated, partial, dissociated or out-of-awareness satisfactions of these needs could occur in the practice of the rituals and devotions. (This provision, with the help of alcohol, probably kept many societies going).

Each society permits the individual freedom to explore certain areas of the world and prohibits certain other explorations by imposing taboos, which in interpersonal terms, as you know, is the not-me, the area of the unthinkable, the dissociated portion of the personality, and indicates that manifestations of interest were dealt with by massive disapproval.

Societies change when the irrational dogmas are put into the light of investigation, bringing the forbidden into awareness. This is essentially the same process that is responsible for change in individuals, in living or in therapy. The scientific era was ushered in about 300 years ago with the release from the limitation of the taboos imposed on curiosity concerning the physical world. The given order was questioned and tremendous energy (aggression) for exploration was released-to the extent that the physicists at least feel they have just about exhausted the field.

In therapy one occasionally encounters an individual who has been depressed and deprived all his life. The first task in such a case is to counter the apathy. How is it you want nothing? What do you want? The next step is to stimulate curiosity-look inside yourself, look outside at the world at others, look at your dreams, your history, and so on.

I want to return to the period of childhood. You will recall that this is the stage when one begins to be trained to become a respectable person according to one's parents' lights. Again, this training goes on in all cultures but we might at this point begin to relate it to recent history.

The training of the child will be by one of two approaches. The first group of parents are the more or less authoritarian. They will be fairly sure of their goals, among which obedience to authority holds the highest priority, and without too much, if any, inner conflict, they unquestionably transmit the idea that life is to be lived as they lived theirs and probably their parents before them. They beat the child into the mold of the past. Curiosity, criticism, and inventiveness are discouraged and dissociated, and the child is on his way to being just like his parents, the respectable silent majority. When the dissociated aspects of his personality are recognized in others, they will be greeted as the embodiment of evil, to be dealt with accordingly. In the juvenile period when he meets his peers, the likelihood is that he will not discover too much difference in them, or in parents and teachers and authority figures. He will subscribe to a rigid, established order of values. The pressure of ostracism and isolation will see to it that his questioning and critical faculties are dissociated, and that threats in this area will be destroyed. As with the inquisition of old, we've had our recent and possibly present inquisitions, and also assassinations of the best advocates of social change.

The other category of parents, whose background is so-called middle class liberal, are those whose children make up the large majority of the group which is the main subject of this paper. These people (the parents) are more open to change themselves. They know there is more than one world-more than the authoritarian world with its certain goals. But they have made their adjustment and found their place in that world, whose values they somewhat deplore. Often they have regretfully compromised the beliefs of their own youth, and compensated for the loss with material preoccupations. Still, they have had a broader experience with two or three generations of partial enlightenment and questioning of the order of things; they are not sure which goals to teach. I think they try to teach both simultaneously or alternately.

How do you tell a child to be open and honest and trusting and feeling in a world where you must learn to be cunning and wily and deceitful to avoid getting hurt? These parents are conflicted and uncertain, knowing that they live in a conflicted world; but they do encourage their children in social criticism, encourage their curiosity and support interests that lead to personality individuation. These parents want their children to be creative. In a word, they raise their children to be a little more advanced than the current level of culture. And these parents could not have done otherwise. They live in a rapidly changing technological world promising plenty, with a juvenile system of production and exchange which at best gives lip service to human needs; they know how the world works. In the home they try to achieve a saner world geared to the actual needs of the children. They thus become identified as "permissive parents." They are the products or victims of their own experience, and yet the inevitable harbingers of change.

Perhaps history will one day accord some honors to them. They have, on the one hand, taught love for fellow man, yet valued the rewards of self-seeking. They have taught learning and enlightenment, but also not to rock the boat. They have said that there is more to living and a better way than the world about you lives, but we have been afraid or unable to live it. In sum, by word and deed they have enlightened their offspring as to the irrationality of their culture as far as human needs are concerned.

And all of this happens in the childhood and juvenile periods. This training, in other words, cannot as yet exert very much influence on the developing juvenile in any personal sense. He is not yet capable of what we call fully human living, but the training facilitates an openness that really takes on significance in the next stage.

At this point we look at youth, and the nature of preadolescent development, which Sullivan has called the quiet miracle. No matter what has transpired before in any juvenile, in all eras of history and all areas of the world there now emerges a powerful new motivation-the need for intimacy. One finds another person of one's own sex, a chum if you please, with whom one can exercise this need. For the first time one finds another person with whom one can have perfectly frank and open communication about all aspects of living without fear of criticism or rebuff. Each of the individuals, for the first time, defers to the needs of the other, and supports the other's self-esteem. In the development till now behavior has been more or less well adjusted self-centeredness. Now the experience is love, which signifies that the needs of the other are at least as important to one as one's own. The nature of the change is such that one begins only now to feel that one belongs to the human race. At the time when Sullivan wrote about it, he felt that for most people it represented the height of human contented living, and that from here on the course was downward. This short period of awareness and enhancement of humanness is rapidly followed by the appearance of pubertal change in the adolescent, and the capacity to experience lust, the development of a need for intimacy with the opposite sex and the patterning of mutually satisfactory sexual relationships, with the concomitant need to take one's place in the adult society.

What is so terribly important to appreciate, in Sullivan's view, is that these developments are rooted in human biological needs and, as such, have the same order of urgency as those referred to when I discussed the infant's experience with deprivation.

In Freud's day and until recently, the interests and behavior of the young were oriented to compete with the father, to displace him, to be better than him-in our view the competitive preoccupations of the juvenile development. The humanistic urges of the preadolescent stage were dissociated, and in their place appeared a "compensatory hardness." When some years ago I taught a course in dreams, from the interpersonal viewpoint, it was possible to demonstrate that many of Freud's own dreams (the Irma dream and the botanical dream as well as others) were derivative of aspects of personality of that period. In other words, he was more human in his dreams, as probably most of us are.

The curious development today is that an expanding group of middle-class youths, who too are driven by the needs of adolescence, do not wish to emulate or displace their elders. Is it possible they are just being difficult? Or could they have something else in mind? After all how many guitar players does a society need? Today there is a large and growing body of youth who are, so to speak, driven by the needs of adolescence and a good part of their behavior expresses an attitude to the larger society that varies from (1) open attack on its institutions, (2) dramatizations-clothes, dress, manners, interests, and behavior-that ridicule the institutions and (3) other behavior which insulates them from the institutions. And along with this are lively experiments in social invention. The gang culture, which was so prominently portrayed in the literature of the thirties and forties, is being displaced   by a larger, somewhat loosely organized youth culture, which seems more and more to stand in opposition to the surrounding culture.

This youth culture is involved in a great deal of social invention in the areas of intimacy and sex, and a coincident testing and protesting of the irrationality of the adult culture. Perhaps these adolescents are too young to be fully wise, though young enough to be adventurous. One senses very strongly in them a certain joylessness and desperation and lostness as if they also knew something about their ultimate future that haunted them.

Personal growth and individuation invariably ensue in a one-to-one relationship; in some sense, the juvenile stage is always an artifact. The child and the juvenile really do not want very much from the environment other than to be allowed to find their self-centered way; they do not understand, and care less, what other people are about. Any divergence from that attitude is a careful adjustment in the interest of security, the forms being strictly reflective of the world one happens to have been born into. But in the adolescent period, the maturing tendencies need the humanness of another. The world of two soon becomes one of three, then four, and societies in miniature spring up in which the care, concern, loyalty, interest, and mutual responsibility of one for the other become the model of possibilities. Fully human status is accorded by one to the other. A nobility of spirit flows freely. The highest value, a new one, is collaboration. What is possible for them now becomes a possibility for the whole world. Youth dreams of utopias, better worlds of human concern, social justice, public good, and public service, of the world as a place for meaningful living unhampered by the greed and meanness which they will shortly encounter. What is wanted is an honorable and meaningful world in which to develop. And let us keep in mind that all of this is "behavior in the interest of need fulfillment" and, in that sense, not different from the infant's behavior, his crying when hungry, except that now the hunger is for human dignity.

At this point the young people come smack up against the world of their elders. The world they need is not there for them. Two main developments are possible. One group, the authoritarian, becomes anxious and dissociates, accepting the religion, if you will, of the elders, and adopting the prevalent values. The other group (our primary interest) cannot do this. The reason is that you cannot dissociate when you know too much. You cannot die gloriously in Vietnam when you clearly perceive how sordid that adventure really is. And you cannot respect the law when it perverts justice, or the government when it ignores its responsibility to the individual, and so on. But curiously you still need to be a citizen; that was going to be your life's work.

And so in interpersonal terms, there is a pressing need like the infant's hunger, the awareness grows, and you experience fear.

Now if you are in the throes of the experience of fear-and I am suggesting that this is what underlies the present upheaval-you have four ways of dealing with this tension. You may try to destroy the cause of the fear, you may try to neutralize it, you may try to escape it (all fairly direct), or you may try to ignore it, a very complex operation such as you employ when you perform that most dangerous of undertakings, crossing a street. If one accepts this notion, it is not too difficult to understand a great deal of the present behavior. Although one needs to hear in mind that symptoms are always over determined, many symptoms can be seen as at least a partial solution to dealing with fear.

Confrontations with institutions can thus be viewed as attempts to destroy or neutralize the source of fear. Interests in astrology, cults, mysticism, and so forth can be regarded as attempts to escape or ignore the fear, as is the current preoccupation with drugs.

And so I arrive at my central thesis. The interpersonal view is that fear called out by the threat of deprivation of human need is the nuclear force underlying the current phenomenon of Youth in Turmoil. In infancy and childhood, the main fear is that of abandonment by parents whose tenderness is essential for the fulfillment of self-centered needs. Our youth suffer similarly from an ill-defined sense of fear of abandonment by the society they so urgently require to achieve their new mutuality needs. They want to be socially useful in a meaningful sense. And although we have always given institutional or lip service to this goal, the aspects of meaningfulness are assuming an interpersonal urgency.

I thought it would be interesting to hear what Sullivan himself had to say on this subject. The following excerpts from his writings (1965) are particularly relevant to the present discussion.

The profligate abandon to exploitation, accidental utilization, or wholly useless wastage, of the human values now within our power to identify, seems, however to be the most fundamental defect of our culture, from which flows most of our other evils. As long as the individual fruits of human evolution are so worthless that they can all be thrown into the same bin to rot or keep whole, as chance dictates, it can scarcely matter if some good human material is ground up in the machinery of law. By the time one now becomes politically significant, he has generally worn himself down to the point at which his formula, his trick of making a living, seems to be about the last thing that he can learn. If it is scrapped by the appearance of a better formula, he may find himself impoverished and his family reduced to want, without hope. It is all "up to" him; life is all a competition, if not a conflict, in which tears are not wasted on the loser. In such a society, we can scarcely expect that the conservation of exceptional human abilities and their untrammeled nurture will become a function of the state.

Whatever his place in the social fabric, the adolescent can scarcely fail to discover in his seeking of a way of life that the satisfaction of some of his tendencies is anything but a simple matter. Mores, law, economic pressures, population concentration and mobility, intercommunication, disintegrative criticism, privilege, privation-above all, the total disintegration of the stable world for which his parents trained him-combine to impress on him the incomprehensibility of life as it goes on around him. He becomes afraid. Moreover, as he seeks to rid himself of fear, he discovers that everyone is afraid, excepting only the stupid. Three paths open before him. His personality organization and his opportunity determine the course that he shall try. He may be able to postpone the plunge, seeking the relative security of the university and the pursuit of knowledge, perhaps having recourse to compensatory dynamics reducing the stress that he experiences. But this is no panacea, for he now embodies tendencies that cannot be discharged in this way. Maladjustments of severe degree are frequent-psychoneuroses, anxiety states, even major psychoses-among those to whom the higher education is primarily a delay in meeting life. He may, particularly if he is enabled by a juvenile personality and the opportunity, adopt the ideal of respectability, and recast himself as rapidly as may be to compliance with the conventional hypocrisies and evasions of his class, making up for the loss of self-esteem by overvaluing material augmentations of his self, and draining off dangerous tensions by a surreptitious "double life," gambling, alcoholic over indulgences, or the pursuit of other excitements that are only partly frustrating-all of which dwarf his potentialities to the level of a solid citizen and fix him in the pattern of late adolescence for life. Or he may identify himself directly or secondarily with a kindred group that lives in some degree of disharmony with the prevailing majority, often somewhat stealthily, coming frequently to waste his youth and energy in misdirected revolt against fantastically exaggerated opposition, in pursuit of poorly-judged goals, or in the overzealous nurture of illusion based on misapprehension of what he seeks. It used to be that generally the adolescent came finally to "settle down"-an expression all the better in that the process was often a regressive disintegration of interest from the adolescent state. The "settling" process has grown quite uncertain, of late, and many factors suggest there will be no return to the good old days. (1965, pp. 219-220).

Until the indissolubly interpersonal character of social life shall have been perceived as a basic feature of every human personality, and the notion of private good is dissipated as an unworkable fiction, there will continue to be increasing disregard both of anachronistic regulation and of the personal necessity of interest in the general welfare. With a more sound psychobiological view, the cultivation of prejudice and the working of personal advantage by playing on prejudice will be regarded as juvenile and unsuited to man's estate. The cultivation of a broad tolerance coupled with a passion for the facts of personality growth and interaction seems to me to offer the only road out of our present impasse in the management of ourselves amongst others. (1965, pp.327-328).

Before concluding I must say a few words about anxiety and my idea of the role it plays in all of this turmoil. Like the need for security, anxiety is always part of the human living, and a complicating factor in interpersonal living. But if, theoretically, we could raise an absolutely anxiety-free adolescent, he would be in the same turmoil as the rest of his group. What he needed would not be attainable because this is the wrong time in history to be self-consciously adolescent. Men hunger for than food.

As a psychiatrist, I can only affirm something that Frieda Fromm- Reichmann says to her patient in Hannah Green's book *I Never Promised You a Rose Garden*. When the patient, a severely ill schizophrenic comes in one day and is behaving somewhat dramatically, Frieda exclaims,

Not only sick, God help us, but adolescent too! . . . Only please help me to see which is the sickness against which we pit our whole strength, and which is the adolescence that is only another sure sign that you are one hundred per cent Earth-one and woman-to-be.

REFERENCES

Green, Hannah. *I Never Promised You a Rose Garden* (New York: Holt, Reinhart, and Winston,1964).
Sullivan, H. S. *The Interpersonal Theory of Psychiatry* (New York: W.W.Norton,1953).
- *Personal Psychopathology*, Washington,D.C. William Alanson White Psychiatric Foundation, 1965).

CHAPTER SIX
ON THE DYNAMICS OF
INTERPERSONAL ISOLATION*

Joseph Barnett

In its naked form, the experience of isolation is most often reported by psychotic patients. The most vivid descriptions of the overwhelming and disorganizing nature of pure isolation have been written by those who have worked most extensively with these patients or by patients themselves. But isolation is not reserved for psychotics. It is a universal experience and is seen constantly in our work with neurotic patients. Indeed, analytic exploration regularly reveals active and organized patterns of isolation-seeking operations in our patients. This paper will explore the dynamics of interpersonal isolation and especially those neurotic needs for isolation, both overt and covert, which I call isolationism. It will seek the roots of such isolation-seeking operations in that organization of experience and meaning we call the self, and therefore its ultimate cause in the development of interpersonal cognition.

Intimacy and isolation are the point and counterpoint of interpersonal relatedness. Both experiences may be defined in relation to the self, and both have important influences on the further growth and integrity of the self.

I would define intimacy as the meaningful integration of self with others. It has its roots in what Sullivan (1953) called the basic human need for tenderness and its evolution in the self. Note that I avoid the narrower usage of the term intimacy which equates it with the acquisition of genital activity, and use instead its general sense as a phase-specific interaction with significant others which grows and changes throughout life. This definition emphasizes the relative and evolving nature of the concept, the connection between the earliest experiences of human contact and tenderness and later developments, and the integral relationship of the concept of intimacy with the self. Intimacy is relative in that it varies with every stage of life with the evolving needs, abilities and capacities of the person, and in that it varies from person to person depending on the nature and integrity of the sense of self. The basic requirement of intimacy is that its participants be known to each other. In turn, this requires both the wish to know, i.e., the interest,

*Presented at Colloquin of New York University Postdoctoral Program in Psychoanalysis and Psychotherapy, November 5, 1976.

effort, and concern, and the decision to be known, i.e., to allow exposure of self to the other. And, if we include, as I do (Barnett, 1968), those states of knowing involved in felt experience as well as syntactically organized experience, i.e., apprehension as well as comprehension, we can extend this basic requirement to all stages in the development of intimacy from infancy on.

In contrast interpersonal isolation may be defined as the real or experienced absence or loss of meaning of the self in relations with significant others. This definition emphasizes the perceived loss of significance and function with others that I feel is central to true isolation. My intent here is to distinguish between isolation and those states of separation in which self or its meaning remain intact. Fromm-Reichmann (1959) felt that we need to develop precision in our concepts of isolation and loneliness, and proposed distinctions between what she called "true loneliness" and loneliness. I suggest that we reserve concepts like loneliness, separateness, estrangement, and alienation to those experiences in which there is either continued presence of the integrity of self and its functions with others, or a change in the sense of self with altered but existing role perceptions. in loneliness and separation, for example, the sense of self usually remains intact, and one experiences one's functions and roles with the absent other, even if only in memory or imagination. Estrangement and alienation, with their implication of becoming strangers, denote a change in perception of self and its roles, often enough neurotic and limiting as Fromm (1941) and Horney (1950) have indicated, but not yet as destructive to the self or as painful as isolation.

The experiences of intimacy and isolation exist as the ongoing dialectic of interpersonal living. They are cognitive experiences, derived from the evolving self and its operational counterpart, the self-system. Both intimacy and isolation, in turn, influence and modify the self. Intimacy is necessary to the growth and integrity of the self and enriches and broadens its operational possibilities. Isolation, on the other hand, is destructive to the self. In that it entails the absence of significance of the self to one's social environment, it causes progressive deterioration of the sense of self, as well as progressive constriction of its operational possibilities.

Let me define at this point my use of the two concepts which I feel are central to the understanding of the dynamics of these phenomena. They are the concepts of self and of self system. The self-system, a term introduced by Sullivan (1953) refers to the developmental organization of interpersonal operations around the gradient of anxiety structured by early experiences. In its development, the self system evolves operational patterns whose aims are to avoid significant amounts of anxiety. It is, in effect, the action template for mental and behavioral operations in the search for gratification of needs in the presence of interpersonal security. The concept of the self-system is an important conceptual tool for the understanding of the relationship between present and past behavior, and of the evolution of the earliest stages of the self.

The self-system alone, however, in my opinion is inadequate to explain the complexity of the self. In interpersonal terms the self may be conceived of as the privately organized recognition of one's interpersonal and social relatedness. It is an essentially cognitive process in that it is the experience, both felt and known, of one's meaning to one's environment especially in terms of one's perception of one's roles and functions. The self has its roots in the early self-system and evolves with the development of cognition. But, as a cognitive system, it develops a life of its own and becomes more complex as additional information and meanings are included through experience. From birth on, a person participates in an implicit dialogue of meaning with his social environment, and the self becomes a repository of ever expanding, complex and often contradictory referents. Not only the experience with anxiety in early interpersonal relations, but all of living contributes, explicitly or implicitly, information about self, others, and the nature of relationships. A person experiences meaning in his interaction with others, in his culture with its social structure, its institutions, its class system, its art, music and dance, its mores, and its religions. He derives assumptions about self from the relations of the sexes, from education, and from his work. These meanings may be directly derived about the self by the reflected appraisals of others or by direct observation. Meanings may also be indirect and external, providing data about the self through such mechanisms as identification or inference making. Meaning systems concerning the self may be accumulated which are contradictory or even at times mutually exclusive, or they may be fragmented and inconsistent. All of these influence the sense of self and eventually the operations that stem from self.

An additional source of meaning centrally important to the development of the self derives from the information and ways of thinking inherent in the belief systems and ideologies implicit in all organized social living. Culture, class, nationalities, politics, religions, science, philosophies, and even families have at least implicit ideological systems and premises which affect meaning and the sense of self and others.

Let us return at this point to the question of isolation and to a problem even more vexing to the practicing analyst than the theoretical complexities. In what seems a paradox, our patients regularly reveal that they seek isolation in open or covert fashion, and do so in such a patterned way that it is evident that these operations are not random, but rather are organized around meaning systems. Why do people choose to pursue isolation? Do they seek the pain and constriction of self inevitable in such a course? Is the explanation for such behaviors to be found solely in the fears of intimacy and the security operations of the patient? I believe not. I believe rather that meanings have been integrated at some level that provide a belief that the best interests of the self are served by some form or forms of isolation from others. Such beliefs, then, are essentially policies of isolationism implicit in that organization of interpersonal experience and meaning we call the self. In other words, isolationism in our patients does not necessarily represent a masochistic position, nor need it represent fears of intimacy, though at times either or both may be the case. More generally, isolationism represents the limited best the patient can conceive of, given his particular assumptions about self, others, and relationships, and his conflicted or impoverished expectations of what interpersonal living has to offer.

The developing self, which involves the person's most private meaning systems, derives in the last analysis from the implicit cognitive matrix of the family, which I have called the family's ideology (Barnett, 1971, 1973). It is the family ideology which forms the structure of meaning that is the source of the person's experience of self, and of the operations of his self- system which maintain and express that experience.

I have used the concept of a family ideology to underscore the existence in the family of implicit cognitive systems-systems of knowing and of meaning as well as systems of innocence-which design the beliefs and experience of the developing child, and are supported and enforced by the family community. The ideology of the family defines the areas of selective attention and inattention-what may be known and what must not be known by its members. It defines the private, shared definitions of experience, the values, preferences, and aversions which form the assumptions of its members. It includes specific dogmas, myths, and taboos which add the weight of authority to central and often shaky assumptions that are necessary to support the family system. It designs the roles of those within the family in terms of functions necessary for maintenance of the system, and even defines the rules for discourse and interaction between its members. The family ideology derives from the interaction of the parents and their need to maintain a homeostasis geared to their needs and selves. It fashions the child's cognitive experience, not only defining his roles and functions, but even designing how he may perceive himself and others. Its special importance lies in the fact that it is the bridge over which personal and cultural belief systems have their confluent impact on the individual.

The family ideology defines the beginnings of the sense of self and its patterns of permissible operations with others. It is here that we must look for the seeds that give rise to policies of isolationism in the developing child whose true needs would be best met in the integration of patterns of intimacy.

Each family ideology generates specific policies of isolationism. In a general sense, these policies derive from the information introduced into the needs, roles, and relationships within the family. Parents who require a personal world ordered along the hierarchical divisions of master and subject, those who need to deny the existence of needs, those who see human warmth as weakness and vulnerability, those who view pleasure as sinful, those who require ambition and success- all these parents structure systems in which the need for intimacy is in conflict with the need for self-esteem, so that isolationist policies are inevitable, In families where significance is connected with performance and achievement, for example, in order to achieve a sense of self, excessive patterns of isolationism motivated by competitiveness and envy are created. In families which idealize secrecy, stoicism, and control of feelings as being strength, those requirements of intimacy such as self-exposure and openness are reduced to weakness. Those family ideologies organized around dependency and service create fears of intimacy as exploitation. Parents who fear individuality, separateness and privacy, create intrusive and controlling systems in which intimacy implies the threat of being invaded or taken over by another. And families that affectively overload their members make intimacy seem like an invitation to a loss of self.

These suggestions must be brief in this presentation, but I hope merely to illustrate the pervasiveness and the determining nature of the family ideology on the patterning both of the fears of intimacy and of policies of isolationism. I have suggested how the family provides the matrix of meaning that determines much of how one sees oneself in relation to the world. Let us now examine more generally the impetus for isolationist tendencies in types of family ideologies.

Families that may be called insular provide one type of impetus for isolationist tendencies. These families are organized around beliefs that the family is especially different, unique, or separate from other families. This "we against the world" belief system usually evolves from especially insecure parents who hope thereby to increase family solidarity. It varies from milder forms of isolation to the severe forms of isolation seen in certain rather paranoid families where suspiciousness and fear are the dominant feeling tones about the extra familial environment. Characteristically, the insular family maintains their system by incessant propagandistic interpretations of the motives of others. Thus if little Jimmy is in conflict with his peers because of his competitiveness, his single minded dedication to performance at school, and his attempts to ingratiate himself with authority by being "class monitor" and authority surrogate, the family's interpretation of the conflict as the hostility of his peers because they are envious of him and his achievements blocks resolution of peer conflict. Unfortunately, this interpretation not only gives Jimmy a rather distorted and propagandistic notion of the meaning of these events, but it also increases his isolation and minimizes his opportunity for learning better how to integrate intimacy with his peers with achievement. The family ideology has managed to polarize intimacy seeking and self-esteem through performance, rather than to aid in integrating them. Family insularity and the ideologies which create and support it, lead inevitably to constriction, intolerance, and hopelessness about the possibility of meaningful collaboration with others.

More usually, the isolationist tendencies bred within families involve the creation of intra familial isolation rather than insularity. Family therapy practice and research has been most helpful in identifying patterns in families which lead to isolation of one or more of the family members. Such patterns as splits and alliances, scapegoating and extrusion (Ackerman, 1958), double-binding (Bateson et al., 1956), and flooding of affect (Barnett, 1968), have been studied in detail as mechanisms which isolate members of the family from each other, and which contribute to role perceptions and the individual's sense of self. Intra familial patterns of isolation are replicated in later life through the sense of self and the self-system. Patients often seem to seek self-definition in terms of the patterns of isolation they experienced within their families of origin. But, e.g., while being the scapegoat may have its rewards within a particular family homeostasis, the larger world rarely offers the same "payoff" for such a role. Intra familial isolation, therefore, creates isolationism around role designs dictated by family injunctions about systems- behavior which is non-integrative and isolating in the extra familial world. Much transference behavior which involves the replication of such isolating systems-behavior is inadequately dealt with in more usual approaches to transference phenomena.

In clinical terms, isolation spans the gamut of normal and pathological living. Discrete policies of isolationism may be found in all of us, constricting our growth and limiting our experiences with others. But in the neuroses, isolationism takes on a darker visage. It is central to the disordered patterns of living, the styles of integrating with others that lead to the increasing spiral of dissatisfactions and insecurities that mark the neurotic personality.

Indeed, theoreticians like Horney (1950), who includes isolation as one of the conditions of basic anxiety, Sullivan (1953), who most succinctly defines the apposition of intimacy and isolation as the root cause of disordered living. Fromm (1941), who emphasizes the terror of isolation in the process of individuation, Angyal (1965), who defines the essence of neurosis as the state of isolation, and Erikson (1959), who indicates the need for social relatedness at each stage of development, have pointed the way to the need for more consistent and penetrating analysis with our patients of their active role in creating the isolation which is, at least implicitly, what troubles them most.

Policies of isolationism are utilized in situations which represent specific threats to either the sense of self or to self-esteem. These threats are woven, through the agency of the family ideology, into the very fabric of the systems of meaning that determine the experience of self. Their potency rests on the fact that threats to the integrity or existence of the self are so intolerable.

Threats to self-esteem are created by the perception that certain patterns of operations with significant others meet with criticism, rejection, ridicule, attack, or belittlement. Isolationism is frequently organized around these experiences of rebuff. In essence, they constitute partial aversion reactions in which there is a renunciation of needs for collaboration with others relative to the degree of anticipated pain.

Threats to one's sense of self are more extreme in their effects. Certain family ideologies minimize or even abort individuality. Their response to intimacy-seeking operations are often those of intrusion or of affective overload. Patients whose parents manifested their anxiety by intrusiveness, experience the possibility of intimacy as potential invasion and loss of self. Those who have experienced inordinately exaggerated affective responses, like rage, seductiveness, and despair, experience reciprocal intimacy as being overwhelmed. Both fear being "taken over" or "being made nothing of" by the other, and their sense of self develops a fortress-like quality in which isolationism is the drawbridge which saves the self from the threatening other. Fear of damage or loss of self is central to the question of what sets isolationism in motion, and at the same time points us towards recognition of the most obvious forms that isolationism may take in response to these threats. Gross attempts at isolating self from others are seen in the common mechanisms of withdrawal, distantiation, and hostile provocation of the environment. Varied forms of isolation have been the subject of much psychoanalytic literature, and I shall not dwell on them. I prefer, rather, to discuss certain fairly common interpersonal dynamisms not usually directly related to this pattern that I consider have their importance primarily as plentiful; the problem involves rather the limited nature or even the total absence of real experience. In the equation of self and other, narcissism effectively eliminates the self, with the other becoming merely audience.

Another form that isolationism frequently takes is the symptom complex we refer to as *depression*. Bonime (1976) has defined depression, accurately I feel, as an interpersonal practice. He considers the dynamics of depression as manipulative attempts both to punish the environment and at the same time to extract one's demands from others. Beck (1967) has underscored, in his work on depression, the cognitive content of attitudes about self and others that is a major part of the syndrome. My own view is consonant with the view of these authors. I feel that depression represents both a form of isolationism and to some extent the felt experience of that isolation. Depression, like narcissism, is a particular form of isolationism and cuts across personality lines. Depression often appears as the end product of other forms and techniques of isolationism, indicating the failure and bankruptcy of the person's learned attempts to achieve security through operations that are essentially isolating. The symptoms of depression are in themselves a vivid portrayal of the person's attempts to isolate himself from others, and to use the insulation of deadness and the anesthesia of affectlessness to ward off the pain as well as the threat of intimacy. The vindictiveness we see in depressed patients is often the only sign of a continued affective tie with others. It serves both to maintain their tenuous relatedness as well as to further coerce the environment to meet the patient's demands. But, as is so typical where policies of isolationism prevail, it too serves only to increase and reinforce isolation. Suicidal thoughts and fantasies are the despairing attempts both to achieve the final isolation as a surcease of pain and despair, and at the same time to achieve the significance to and response from others for which the patient so hopelessly yearns.

Another covert form of isolationism which occurs often among young adults as well as older populations is the *creation of systems of idealization and disillusionment*. I find this a rather frequent pattern of preventing intimacy and significant contact with a real other, and of seeking and maintaining isolation. There are some patients who repeatedly relate to significant people in their lives, such as their parents or children with such a degree of idealization that it is clear that meaningful contact and true intimacy are excluded as possibilities. Intimacy requires mutual knowledge and exposure, and the essence of idealization is that fantasy obscures reality and blurs knowledge. The isolating person, in effect, wipes out the other by substituting his own needs and fantasies for the reality of the other.

Idealization always exists on the brink of its other face, disillusionment, which is invariably catastrophic to even the pretense of the relationship. The frequency with which this pattern, of idealization followed by disillusionment, occurs in some patients should make us suspect and interpret the existence of a distinctly patterned policy of isolationism, and to relate it to the integrity of the self and its conceptual anlage.

Quite common in our society is a form of isolationism that can be called *the conventionalization of experience*. In this pattern, personal meaning is avoided in interpersonal relations, and conventional forms are substituted. It is a form of "keeping up with the Jones's," in terms not of external possessions but rather in terms of operations usually defined by the self-interpersonal behavior, experiences of relatedness, and social responses to others. Those who use this form of isolationism have little sense of self and are often childish and immature personalities. Their deadness and lack of imagination are striking. They are divorced from truly personal wants and wishes, and substitute instead what they feel they are supposed to do, feel, and want. Their inner emptiness and lack of sense of self effectively isolates them from organizing meaning in interpersonal experiences and makes them particularly prone to use external belief-systems and ideologies to define themselves. Their isolation, moreover, is so well denied and rationalized by their childish involvement with conventional forms that they often claim to have been totally unaware of their isolation for many years until specific traumata cause retrospective reevaluation. Usually quite refractory to insight and introspection, they may experience their isolation due to events that demand a rapid change in role perceptions, as, for example, when a "happy marriage" of 15 years duration suddenly collapses, or when a "typical family" suddenly erupts into delinquency or psychosis.

A pattern of isolationism related to that of conventionalization of experience, but worth separate consideration, is that of *pseudo-intimacy*. Pseudo-intimacy is a form of relatedness in which the person assumes intimate relatedness with the other because some component aspect of intimacy exists, but actually excludes the possibility of integrating many areas with a whole person. Sexual involvement, mutual exhibitionism, identical occupations and professions, shared secrets, or membership in exclusive clubs, organizations, or ideological groups are among the forms that pseudo-intimacy make take. Common to all is the exclusion of knowledge, sharing or mutual fulfillment of needs except in a narrow but personal area. Pseudo-intimacy derives both from the classical intrapsychic mechanism of isolation of affect from ideation, and from family patterns of pseudo-mutuality described by Wynne et al. (1958). These, then, are some of the most common covert manifestations of individual policies of isolationism. I have tried to be representative and touch on the most important forms of isolationism, to sketch a rationale rather than attempt to be all-inclusive. My hope is primarily to indicate the presence, the potency, and the interpretive significance of isolationism in our attempts to understand and aid the nonproductive living in which most of our patients are imbedded. I believe that the experience of isolation and those patterns and policies of isolationism that evolve in the person's development are central issues that must be resolved by all of us. They are related to the development of cognition as well as to the development and integrity of the self. Indeed, one might say that the study of isolationism is the study of those organizations of meaning and behavior that prevent us from becoming fully human.

References

Ackerman, N. W. (1958), *The Psychodynamics of Family Life*, Basic Books,Inc., New York.

Angyal, A. (1965), *Neurosis and Treatment: A Holistic Theory*, John Wiley and Sons, Inc., New York.

Barnett, J. (1968), Cognition, thought, and affect in the organization of experience, *Science and Psychoanalysis*, Vol. XII, J. Masserman (Ed.), Grune and Stratton, New York, 237- 247.

Barnett, J. (1971), Dependency conflicts in the young adult, *Psychoanalytic Review*, 58(1), 111-125.

Barnett, J. (1972), Therapeutic intervention in the dysfunctional thought processes of the obsessional, *Am. J. Psychother.*, 26(3), 338-351.

Barnett, J. (1973), On ideology and the psychodynamics of the ideologue, *J. Am. Acad. Psychoanal*, 1(4),381-395.

Bateson, G., D. Jackson, J. Haley, and J. H. Weakland (1956), Toward a theory of schizophrenia, *Behav. Sci., 1*, 251-264.

Beck, A. T. (1967), *Depression*, Harper and Row, New York.

Bonime, W. (1959), The psychodynamics of neurotic depression, *American Handbook of Psychiatry*, S. Arieti (Ed.), Basic Books, New York, 239-255.

Forrest, T. (1974), The family dynamics of maternal violence, *J. Am. Acad. Psychoanal*, 2(3), 215-230.

Fromm, E. (1941), *Escape from Freedom*, Rinehart and Co., New York.

Erikson, E. H. (1959), Identity and the life cycle, in *Psychological Issues*, Pt.

1, International Universities Press, New York.
Fromm-Reichmann, F. (1959), On loneliness, in *Psychoanalysis and Psychotherapy: Selected Papers of Frieda Fromm-Reichmann*, D. M. Bullard (Ed.), University of Chicago Press, 325-336.
Horney, K. (1950), *Neurosis and Human Growth*, W. W. Norton and Co., New York.
Sullivan, H. S. (1953), *The Interpersonal Theory of Psychiatry*, W. W. Norton and Co., New York.
Wynne, L. C. Ryckoff, I. M., Day, J., and Hirsch, S. 1. (1958), Pseudo-mutuality in the family relations of schizophrenics, *Psychiatry, 21*, 205-220.

CHAPTER SEVEN
IDENTIFICATION AND
SOCIALIZATION
IN ADOLESCENTS

Donald Meltzer

Surely, it will be said- and- rightly-the analytic consulting room, in its heat of infantile intimacy, is not the place to study the social behavior of adolescents. But it can, through clarification of the internal processes-of motivation and expectation, identification and alienation-throw a special and unparalleled light upon social processes to aid the sociologist, educator, psychiatrist, and all those persons of the adult community whose job it is to preserve the boundaries of the adolescent world and foster the growth and development of those still held within its grip.

Our times reveal more clearly than other historical periods the truth of the existence of an "adolescent world" as a social structure, the inhabitants of which are the happy-unhappy multitude caught betwixt the "unsettling" of their latency period and the "settling" into adult life, the perimeter of which may not unreasonably be defined, from the descriptive point of view, as the establishment of mating and child rearing. From the metapsychological point of view of psychoanalysis, stripped as it is of social and moral evaluation, this passage from latency to adulthood may be described most forcefully in structural terms, whose social implications this paper is intended to suggest.

The developmental pathways which traverse this world of adolescence lead from splitting in the self to integration, in relation to objects which, also by integration, are transformed from a multitude of part-objects to a family of whole objects in the internal world. Upon this model the external relationships *must* be regulated. As long as splitting in self and objects is still considerable, the experience of self will be highly fluctuating, depending on the dominance of one or other of the three types of psychic experience of identity in consciousness *(see below)*. In a sense one may say that the *center of gravity* of the experience of identity shifts-and in the adolescent it shifts wildly and continually.

This phenomenon, the continual shifting of the center of gravity of the sense of identity, produces the characteristic quality of emotional instability seen in adolescence and since it is based on the underlying splitting processes, the varying states of mind are in very little contact with one another. Hence the adolescent's gross incapacity to fulfill commitments to others, to carry through resolutions of his own or to comprehend why he cannot be entrusted with responsibilities of an adult nature. He cannot fully experience that the person who did not fulfill and the person who undertook to fulfill the commitment were the same person, namely himself. He therefore feels a continual grievance of the "brother's keeper" type.

His solution to this terrible state is a flight into group life where the various parts of himself can be externalize into the various members of the "gang." His own role becomes simplified greatly, though not completely, for status and function in the group is in flux to a certain extent. This flight-to-the-group phenomenon is even in effect evidently dynamically in the adolescent who is not a member of any gang, for, by being the "pariah," he fulfills a role which the gang formation requires, that of the totally alienated psychotic part of the personality of those who are integrated in the gang. The isolate in turn projects his own more healthy parts.

I would remind you that this is not a descriptive definition of an age group but a metapsychological description of personality organization typical of this age group, though we may meet "latency" in a fifty-year old and adolescence at nine, structurally. The most important fact to be kept in mind in the following discussion is the transition of excessive and rigid splitting in latency, through the fluidity of adolescence as a matrix from which the more orderly and resilient splitting and differentiation of adult personality organization are fashioned.

The *experience of identity* is complex in structure and various in duality. Its unconscious basis we express by the concept of "identification," on the one hand, and the experience of "self," on the other. It contains both characterological and body-image facets and must be taken, *in toto*, as a summation of momentary states of mind, an abstraction of highly variable integration-from individual to individual-from moment to moment. The *experience of identity* also cannot exist in isolation, but only as foreground to the world of objects, internal and external-and to the laws of psychic anti external reality.

There are three types of experiences which carry the feeling of identity, the experience of a part of the self, of identification with an object by introjection, and of identification with an object by projection. These three have a very distinctive quality, one from the other. The experience of a part of the self carries a feeling of limitation akin to littleness, tinged with loneliness. Introjective identification contains an aspirational element, tinged with anxiety and self-doubt. But the state of mind achieved by projective identification is fairly delusional in its quality of completeness and uniqueness. The attendant anxieties, largely claustrophobic and persecutory, are held very separately in the mind from the identity experience.

I wish to come back now to the more central problem, the underlying severe confusion at all levels with which the adolescent is contending. As I have said, with the breakdown of the obsessional, rigid, and exaggerated splitting characteristic of latency structure, an uncertainty in regard to the differentiations internal-external, adult-infantile, good-bad, and male-female which was characteristic of the pre-Oedipal development reappears. In addition, perverse tendencies due to confusion of erogenous zones, compounded of confusion between sexual love and sadism, take the field. This is all "in order," as it were; the group life presents a modulating environment vis-a-vis the adult-world and distinct from the child-world, well equipped to bring this seething flux gradually into a more crystallized state-if the more psychotic type of confusion of identity due to massive projective identification does not play too great a role. To illustrate this I will describe two cases briefly.

But first to clarify the concept. Where the reappearance of masturbation [4] brings with it a strong tendency, driven by infantile oral envy, to abandon the self and seize an object's identity by intrusion into it, the stage is set for a type of confusional anxiety which all adolescents experience to some extent. This confusion centers on their bodies and appears with the first pubic hair, the first breast growth, first ejaculation, and so forth. Whose body is it? In other worlds, they cannot distinguish with certainty their adolescent state from infantile delusions-of-adulthood induced by masturbation with attendant projective identification into internal objects. This is what lies behind the adolescent's slavish concern about clothes, make-up and hair style, hardly less in the boys than in the girls.

Where this mechanism is very strongly operative and especially where it is socially "successful," the building up of the "false self," of which Winnicott has spoken, takes place.

Case Material

Rodney entered analysis at eighteen after the complete academic failure of his first year at university. He was, two years later, able to regain a place and continue his education, but scholastic failure soon appeared as the least of his difficulties. His latency period had been built on a severe split in his family adjustment, as he had been a devoted, endlessly helpful and unfailingly polite son among the otherwise rather stormy children. In fact, in his own eyes he was never a child but a father-surrogate [4,5] in all matters other than sexuality. To compensate, he appropriated as his due an absolute privacy and self-containment which, with the onset of puberty, became converted into a cover of absolute secrecy for a florid, delinquent bisexual life, while his family behavior remained unchanged- now he was a "manly chap" instead of a "manly little chap."

In dividing himself among his gang he retained as his "self" the worst, most envious and cynical bit of himself. Consequently his relation to others tended to be both forceful and corrupting. The "good" parts of himself tended to remain projected into younger siblings, from whom he maintained a severe, protective distance.

More delusional states of identity occurred relatively infrequently and only under special circumstances-if he were driving his mother's car, or entertaining friends in an outbuilding he had been given as a study. These states could be dangerous indeed, physically and morally, but were soon recognized in the analysis and could be avoided. The re-establishment of contact with good parts, in a therapeutic alliance with the analyst and with internal objects, could take place. Progress was steady and rewarding.

Paul, on the other hand, had entered analysis in pre-puberty because of severe character restriction, with obsessional symptoms, nocturnal rituals, obvious effeminacy-all of which had existed for years but worsened by the break-up of the parents' marriage. The first period of analysis with another analyst utilizing play technique had been virtually non-verbal. In those sessions, he had been preoccupied with painting and art, producing a few pictures analyzable in content but mainly endless preparations-for-painting consisting in mixing colors, making color charts -in fact, concretely being daddy's artist-penis preparing the semen for the coming intercourse. As his symptoms lessened and his school adjustment and work improved, he broke off the analysis, returning to it only three years later when, after passing his O-levels* and working his way to the position of vice-captain of his school, he found himself confronted with A-levels** for which he was totally unprepared.

What had happened in the intervening time was this: The building up of the school-self of athlete-artist-vice captain had become totally time-consuming. It had to be compensated for by a gradual retrenchment from all

---

* Ordinary-level of the G.C.E. (General Certificate of Education)
** Advanced-level of G.C.E. for University entrance.

academic subjects requiring thought or exact knowledge, in favor of those he felt to require talent or to be based on vague statistics. He had become unable to study, but at home or in school consumed his time in the busy-work of preparations or the posturing of absorption-preoccupied always by the fantasies of his appearance in the eyes of others. His paranoia, particularly in relation to laughter, had to be hidden and his own mocking laugh, irreproachably tolerant in timbre, kept a steady stream of projection of feelings of humiliation penetrating into others.

Analytic work to gather together the infantile parts of himself into the transference and to differentiate the delusions-of-adulthood from his true adult personality was most tedious uphill work. Every separation brought a renewed flight into projective identification, represented in dreams by intruding into gardens, climbing into houses, leaving the main road for a trackless swamp, and so forth. Take a typical Friday, for instance. In the Thursday session he had experienced a reawakening of gratitude toward- his mother for providing the analysis, along with guilt about the motor scooter he had insisted on having and the hours of analysis he had missed or wasted. This had been the unusually strong positive reaction to analysis of a dream which showed clearly that the preponderance of his infantile parts wanted analysis, not masturbation, as manifest by the crowd at a school dance sitting at tables demanding food rather than going into the ballroom to dance. By Friday, however, he could whip himself into a state of arrogant contempt for the analysis because the analyst, unlike his art teacher, who had said that a new picture was the first to show a style of his own rather than mimicry of others' styles, did not realize that Paul had now finally emerged from the chrysalis of "student." Relentlessly, then, he would spend the week end mixing paints.

Now note that Paul presented a facade of social integration-the school captain-while Rodney seemed delinquent, corrupted, and isolated from society. But in fact, closer scrutiny shows that Rodney had a gang in which his identity was disseminated and from which it could be retrieved, while Paul had only "friends" who were his enforced colleagues while he was vice-captain and later captain of the school. In fact he was isolated-"well-liked"-to use the immortal phrase of Willy Loman in Arthur Miller's "Death of a Salesman."

These two cases are intended to show the important role of the group as a social pattern in adolescence, indicating that, no matter how delinquent or antisocial it may appear vis-a-vis the adult world, it is a holding position in relation to the splitting foster the gradual lessening of the splitting, diminution of the omnipotence and amelioration of the persecutory anxiety by achievement in the real world.

We must, however, turn back to our analytic experience at the other pole of the adolescent process to comprehend the basis of this dissemination. Experience in carrying latency children into puberty during analysis reveals this in a brilliant way which I will describe through a third case.

Juliet had come to analysis at the age of seven for deeply schizoid character difficulties which rendered her doll-like in appearance and demeanor, utterly submissive to excellent but highly idealized parents. This facade was broken in two areas, explosions of fecal smearing on rare occasions and a witchlike hegemony over a younger sister and her little friends.

Six years of the most arduous analytic work broke through this, enabling her true femininity, artistic talents, and rich imagination to emerge by the time of her menarche. But her masculinity formed the basis of her social adaptation to peers, as shown by the formation of a gang of five girls, all intelligent, attractive, and athletic, who became the "troublemakers" of her girl's school. The general pattern of a very revealing dream of that time was subsequently repeated, again and again. She seemed in the dream, to be one of five convict men who were confined in a flimsy structure made of slats at the top of a tall tree. But every night they escaped and prowled about the village, returning unbeknown to their captors before dawn.

This dream could be related to earlier material regarding masturbatory habits in which her fingers, in bed at night, explored the surfaces and orifices of her body, often accompanied by conscious adventuresome fantasies.

Two years later, when her femininity had established itself in the social sphere as well, she attended her first unchaperoned party, where the boys were somewhat older, drinking occurred, and sexual behavior became rather open. To her surprise she behaved with a coolness and provocativeness which earned her the shouted epithet of "frigid tart" from a boy whose attempt to feel under her skirt she had skillfully repulsed.

That night she dreamed that five convicts were confined to a wooden shed from which they were released by a bad squire on condition that they would steal fruit from the women with fruit stalls in the village and bring the loot to him.

Here one can see that the delinquent organization of the masculine masturbating fingers had been projected into the boys of the party by her "frigid tart" behavior. The fact that the fantasies acted out were infantile and pregenital (anal and oral) was clearly indicated by the stealing of food, a theme well known from the earlier years of analytic work.

This masturbatory theme, the personification of the fingers, seems in fact to turn up with extraordinary frequency in our analytic work and would lead us to the expectation that the typical "gang" of the adolescent would tend, by unconscious preference, to contain five members, or multiples of this number. In other terminology we might say that the gestalt of the adolescent gang would tend most strongly to "close" at five members.[5]

SUMMARY

In this brief paper I have tried to outline some of the knowledge gained by recent analytic experience with children carried into puberty and adolescents carried into adult life. This work was conducted within the framework of theory and technique which is an extension of the developments in psychoanalysis associated with the name of Melanie Klein. It draws very heavily on her delineation of the pregenital Oedipus conflicts,[1] the role of splitting processes in development,[2] and the phenomenology of projective identification as a dynamic mechanism.[2,3] It may not be readily comprehended without a general understanding of her work. The most lucid description of this will be found in Hanna Segal's book.[6]

The thesis has been exemplified, that the return of severe splitting processes, characteristic of infancy and early childhood, which attends the adolescent flux, requires externalization in group life so that the omnipotence and confusional states precipitated by the return of masturbation at puberty may be worked through. The implications for sociological comprehension of the "adolescent world" as a social institution are apparent:

1. Individual psychotherapeutic work should be directed toward the isolated individual, to promote the socialization of his conflicts.

2. The "gang" formation of adolescents needs to be contained in its antisocial aspects but not to be intruded upon by adult guidance.

3. The emergence of individuals from adolescence into adult life is facilitated by measures which lessen the conflict between the sexual aspirations toward mating and other areas of ambition.

REFERENCES

1. Klein, M., "The Oedipus Complex in the Light of Early Anxieties," in

Contributions to Psychoanalysis (London: Hogarth Press, 1945).
2. -." Notes on some Schizoid Mechanisms," in *Developments in Psycho-Analysis* (London: Hogarth Press, 1946).
3. -, *Envy and Gratitude* (London: Tavistock, 1957).
4.   Meltzer, D., "The Relation of Anal Masturbation to Projective Identification," *Int. J. Psychoanal.*, 47 (1966), 335.
5. -, *The Psycho-analytical Process* (London: Tavistock, 1967).
6.   Segal, H., *Introduction to the Work of Melanie Klein* (London: Heinemann, 1964).

CHAPTER EIGHT
SOME CAUSES OF DELINQUENCY

August Aichhorn

Although we must guard against generalization, our study of several cases seems to justify the formulation of a general principle. Delinquency represents one of the departures from the normal in psychic processes, and for this reason a solution of the problem of delinquency depends on understanding the psychic content. Since we have learned to think psychoanalytically, we know that dissocial behavior is the result of disturbed psychic patterns, of abnormal accumulation of affect. The manner in which the psychic energy is utilized determines the direction in which the individual develops: whether he will be psychically normal, whether he will be subjected to nervous illness, or whether he will become dissocial.

Since our explanations and conclusions up until now seem obvious, you may underestimate the necessity for a thorough study of psychoanalysis. You may even believe that you can simply adopt a few psychoanalytic principles and carry on your work as formerly. Such an idea would lead you into dilettantism, which is more dangerous than complete ignorance. Not every delinquent is an interesting psychoanalytic or neurotic problem, but there are so many possible determinants for every delinquent act that our investigation must be guided by sound theoretical knowledge. I do not wish to alarm you, but simply to warn you that unless we avoid all haste and superficiality, we are doomed to failure.

The [following] case is that of an 18-year-old boy brought to me by the mother. My first advice was that the child should be examined by, a psychiatrist. The doctors were unable to find any sign of nervous disorder and attributed the laziness and aggressive behavior of which the mother complained to a conflict within the family. The mother was a widow: the father, who had been foreman in a large factory, had died many years before. After his death, the mother secured an office position which barely sufficed to support herself and the children. The situation had been better during the past year since the oldest daughter had begun to work. She was a year younger than our patient, had learned the trade of seamstress, and was employed in a dress making shop. There were three more children in the family: girls, aged 15, 13, and 10 years.

When the mother resumed with her son after the doctors' examination, I asked her to wait while I interviewed the boy alone. The boy made a feminine impression: he seemed shy and ill at ease, and was at first uncommunicative. It was hard to believe that this boy was capable of the aggressive acts ascribed to him, and I realized at once that they must be momentary outbursts of affect rather than the expression of a brutal nature. I learned the following important facts during the long interview with the boy. He had completed the seventh grade of the public school with a creditable record. His plan to continue his work in high school was interrupted by the death of his father. He wanted to apprentice himself to a painter, but since he could find no opening, he had taken the job of errand-boy in a drug store about December of the same year. Because of his mother's eagerness to have him learn a trade, he gave up this job after a few weeks and apprenticed himself to a carpenter. He liked this job and remained over a year until he discovered that his employer was not a master carpenter and therefore had no right to train apprentices. He was so much annoyed by this that for some time he refused to enter another carpenter shop. Finally, however, he secured another apprenticeship through his mother. He lost this job nine months later because the firm went bankrupt. By this time he had enough of carpentry. His mother tried everything from kind words to beating to make him change his mind, but to no avail. He had no further interest in learning a trade, and after weeks of job-hunting became an errand boy again, this time in a paper store. He was discharged after six weeks because he refused to carry out an order which was offensive to him. A relative now took him in charge because his mother would have nothing more to do with him. He left home to become an apprentice in a planing mill, but returned after eight weeks. Previously there had been only short intervals between jobs, but this time he remained unemployed for half a year. He was brought to me after he had failed to hold his last job, as errand-boy in a dry-goods store.

The boy declared that he did not want to be a burden to his mother since he was strong and healthy, but he refused to become a common laborer as his mother wished. He would be content to learn carpentry if he could be given credit for his first year's apprenticeship, but nobody was willing to straighten out the affair. During the time he was unemployed, he had enjoyed helping his mother with the house. work. He especially liked washing dishes and housecleaning. He read a lot in his spare time-anything that came to his hand, without discrimination. He became excited when we discussed his relationship to the different members of the family. He seemed especially to hate his oldest sister. I learned that his fits of anger were chiefly directed against her. He felt insulted because his sisters belittled him and laughed at him. The oldest sister was the leader in this, and his mother, instead of standing up for him, took the side of the girls. He explained to me with considerable affect that the boy in a family ought to have a say as well as the girls. He liked his mother best, and the sisters in the order of their age, the youngest first. He could not bear his oldest sister because she was always disagreeable and wanted to boss everything. The sisters were quite different in appearance. The oldest was taller than he, had a narrow face, blue eyes, and blond hair. She resembled the mother, but the other sisters looked more like their father. The mother and sisters were very religious, but he had liberal socialistic views, which he had never discussed with his family. They associated only with strict Catholics. They took him to social gatherings with them without knowing how repugnant this was to him. He did not dare tell his mother of the conflict about the difference in their ideas. He liked to visit one of his mother's friends because he met a girl there whom he admired very much although the rest of the people were uncongenial. He was embarrassed when I asked him whether he had ever liked any girls before, but then admitted that at 13 he had been in love with one of his oldest sister's schoolmates who spent a great deal of time with them. He remembered her as similar in appearance to his sister except that her hair was a deeper blond, and her eyes gray-blue. When I asked him whether he was in love at the moment, he blushed, but then spoke with enthusiasm of the girl already mentioned. Had he ever kissed her? "A boy doesn't do that," he replied, flushing and embarrassed. His description of her made her in every way the older sister's opposite, although he seemed unaware of this fact. She had black hair and dark-brown eyes. When I asked whether he knew anyone in his childhood with such eyes and hair, he mentioned his youngest sister.

Questioned about his childhood, he gave several recollections. The first was about "saying pieces" on holidays, an important custom in the family. One time when he was very little, he and his oldest sister had competed in reciting birthday greetings. The father had promised a picture book to the one who recited best. She got the prize, and he was so angry that he tore up the book. The narrative sequence of this incident was reversed in his memory; he began by describing how his father had whipped him for his naughtiness. He also told me that he and this sister had loved to play father and mother as children, and that the youngest sister was always their child in this game.

This ended our interview and I called the mother in. She was irritated that she had been kept waiting, and immediately told me that she could not understand why I had to talk so long to the boy because I knew already what the trouble was; she had told me that at our first meeting before I sent her to the clinic. It was obvious that she felt her authority threatened. She was a lean woman of middle height with sharp features and hard eyes. She gave the impression of being an energetic person whom nothing could daunt. Life had treated her badly from childhood. Although married life had given her material security, she had not had a satisfactory relation~hip with her husband. After his death it had been a struggle to maintain the five children. Her oldest daughter was an exceptional girl who turned over all her earnings to the mother. With her help they could have got along much better if it had not been for the trouble with the boy. The mother felt that her husband never understood the deeper needs of her nature. He was a cheerful person who took life lightly; he was undiscriminating in all his pleasures, including women. There were no open quarrels between them, but the wife withdrew more and more from her husband. "I always had to stand apart from life. My religious upbringing was very strict. When I later discovered how much these principles were contradicted by actual life, I suffered for years until I finally reached a solution within myself."

She spoke of her son in a deprecating way as though he no longer meant anything to her. "He is not a man, just a stupid, stubborn boy who thinks he knows it all. He tries to lord it over his sisters, and naturally they won't stand for it. He carries on so and talks so foolishly that the girls laugh at him; this makes him furious and he attacks them like a wild animal, especially the oldest. If I don't get him out of the house, something terrible is bound to happen. He obeys me; he doesn't dare defy me because he knows that I would whip him even though he is 18 years old. He acts like a child. After he has been up to something, he is very obedient and cleans up everything around the house nicely. He is a very orderly boy; his closet is much neater than any of his sisters', and he gets mad if they disturb anything. On the other hand, he is careless about his person. I have to make sure that his neck and ears are clean. But he will stand before the mirror for an hour arranging his tie and combing his hair. Of course his sisters are annoyed by this. He thinks only of himself. In the morning he won't get up and doesn't clean his shoes. He has no initiative; housework and reading books are no work for a grown boy; he ought to have a steady job. I won't support him any longer. I haven't the money and he has to learn that we won't slave for him. He is not even honest; when I send him to the store, he cheats me in small amounts, which he spends on candy like a school child. I refuse to bear it any longer; he has to take work as a laborer and earn his own bread and butter."

We feel that the mother's complaints are to some extent justified and that she is wise in seeking help in this intolerable situation. What is to be done? Perhaps you think that having heard both sides, we should now bring mother and son together and try to find a middle I road out of the difficulty, encourage one or the other, urge them to be more patient and so try to reach a compromise. *Such a type of procedure would be as ineffectual as a moral lecture about delinquency.* It is not our job to make peace, nor to judge the boy, but I rather to solve the problem. We know that we must first discover the cause of the dissocial behavior by understanding the psychic situation which produced it. For the moment it is only the emotional reaction of this dissocial boy which interest us, and therefore we must examine the facts for their subjective rather than objective validity. Everything we learn about the case must contribute to this. This implies that we take the side of the boy. Since we believe that all psychic manifestations are somehow predetermined, we must say to ourselves, "He is in the right, there must be reasons for this behavior." What would we gain by being shocked, or by joining the ranks of those who are distressed by his behavior? Moral or ethical condemnation will not help us.

The most disagreeable of the boy's traits, his brutality at home and especially that toward the oldest sister, should be our first interest. We eliminate all moral judgments and see the brutality for what it is, the manifestation of a long latent situation. Dynamically this could be expressed by saying that the discharge of psychic energy no longer remains within social bounds. This trait might be constitutionally determined. If we believed this, it would concern us no further; his laziness would be the only problem left for us to deal with. But this can hardly be a case of constitutional brutality since nothing about the boy corresponds to the type-neither the impression he made on me nor the description supplied by the mother. What the boy said made us feel that his aggressions were momentary outbreaks of affect, and as such they deserve our interest. We find aggression directed chiefly against the oldest sister and we have further evidence that he hates her. One of his childhood memories might indicate a source of this hate. As a very small boy, he probably experienced very painful slights. You will remember the story about the birthday book. Experience in the treatment of neurotics by psychoanalysis has taught us that such a memory usually serves as the facade for many other similar memories which are recalled in the course of treatment. We feel that his father was tactless in his treatment of the boy, that he disregarded his feelings and apparently did not understand him. It seems probable, too, that there was actual favoritism shown the little girl by the father. We might therefore say that the boy's dislike of his several sisters was founded on the slights endured as a child, and that he particularly hated the oldest sister because she was her father's favorite. The constellation in this family is one we frequently encounter. The father prefers the daughters to the son, the mother has no special need for affection, and the son is therefore cheated. The same can be true of girls if the situation is reversed.

At this point a few general statements are pertinent. Anyone who has contact with children, whether as parent or teacher, will find himself continually faced with a phenomenon which no effort on his part can quite eliminate. The harmony of every nursery is continually disturbed by feelings of envy and jealousy within the group, though the parents try to avoid any show of favoritism. Observation should have taught us what psychoanalysis has to say on this subject, i.e., that every child regards his brothers and sisters as competitors in the struggle for the important first place in the love of the parents. This rivalry does not endanger the child's development if parents deal sensibly with each situation as it comes. Many mothers do the right thing by instinct; others make continual mistakes without realizing it. In these cases it often happens that the relationship between brother's and sisters lacks warmth even in later life. The more unfavorable the circumstances the greater the likelihood that they will lead to delinquency. The situation of this boy must have been thoroughly unfavorable. In addition to an unsympathetic father he had a clever but hard woman as a mother. Nevertheless we cannot accept his suffering from lack of love as the cause of his delinquency. Why not? Because the other incident which he related about his childhood makes this theory untenable.

We heard that the sister he now hated had at one time been his favorite playmate. This would have been impossible had they been bitter rivals. We might suppose that the relationship had been ambivalent were it not that they played mother and father, with the youngest sister as their child. Of course we do not know how long this relationship between the children lasted, but we are safe in supposing that countless other memories similar in character lie behind the one he told us. Can this fact help us to find a cause for his delinquency? We might set up as a premise the supposition that his hate of his sister was determined by an unconscious erotic tie to her. Because of your lack of familiarity with psychoanalysis, it may sound fantastic to hear talk of an erotic tie where only violent hate manifests itself. If our supposition were founded only on the childhood memory it would have little justification. There are other facts, however, which support this. You may wonder that we should proceed on such a doubtful assumption, especially since psychoanalytic experience teaches us that the first statements of a patient are often altered or refuted by the deeper material which is disclosed later in the analysis. But do not forget that our work differs from that of the psychoanalyst. We are not in the position of being able to wait; because we must act quickly, we are forced to form a picture of a situation after a few interviews. We know that our conclusions are no more than partly right, and that only the result of the treatment will show how far our assumptions were correct. We can lessen the uncertainty by a careful study of the material at our command.

Before returning to the case under discussion, we should make clear what we mean by "erotic tie." We are justified in supposing that the brother and sister shared an intense experience while playing the game of father and mother. We know that this childish game is not always harmless, that children put more into it than is commonly supposed, and that playing husband and wife frequently ends with examining each other's bodies and thus satisfying childish curiosity. We have often found in our practice that children act out in these games what they have observed their parents doing. Under crowded living conditions, it frequently happens that children have the opportunity to see sexual intercourse between their parents. Certainly such games are a source of excitement which can only be termed sexual, although this word is used in a broader sense than usual. The memories which survive these experiences serve to bind the partners strongly to each other, and the more intense the emotion the stronger the tie. Even though he is not caught in the act, the child is certain to learn that what he did and felt on these occasions was wrong. He understands the difference between these games which he invents for his own pleasure and those which are approved. If the drive toward the instinctual pleasure remains stronger than his fear of punishment, the games are continued; if the other impulse conquers, the experience is repressed. Children at this age are not capable of solving the conflict consciously by rejecting the forbidden pleasure. They try therefore to forget the game and everything associated with it, including the feelings for the partner involved, which represent the greatest danger to renewed temptation. Repression cuts these impulses off from this form of expression, but they continue to exist in the unconscious. After conscious control has been lost, these impulses are subjected to the influence of other forces in the unconscious and the result is what the psychoanalyst calls a fixation. We can easily understand that the ties to the child partner are not broken but simply displaced, i.e., an unconscious erotic tie is formed. The danger of this attachment becoming conscious is lessened if the feeling is completely reversed, if the love relationship finds conscious expression as hate. We know have a general conception of what we mean by an unconscious erotic tie, although it is hardly possible to grasp the full significance of this psychoanalytic principle at once. In the case of our patient, we lack proof that the boy's hate for his sister was so determined. If we say that it could have developed out of their childish game, we draw an analogy with the neurotic. But our boy is a delinquent and not a neurotic. We must therefore find other material to strengthen our supposition. I believe it will be helpful to discuss another theory before returning to the facts of the case.

You are familiar with the term puberty. The common belief is that it refers only to the physiological changes, the maturing of the genital organs in both sexes which takes place during this period. But many individuals are unable to fulfill the function of reproduction in spite of having normally developed sexual organs. They are incapable of feeling the necessary attraction for persons of the opposite sex, or else their psychic constitution is such that it demands other than normal sexual gratification. Freud has shown us that an understanding of puberty is impossible unless the psychological component is considered. He has deepened our insight into that psychic development which normally ends with adolescence and has studied the results of disturbances at various points. one fact is of immediate importance to us; that at adolescence the youth should give up his first love objects within the family and replace them by others outside this circle. in psychoanalytic terms the infantile libidinal ties must be loosened in order to free the libido for object relationships outside the family. If the libidinal ties to the objects are too strong, are fixated, it becomes difficult or impossible to loosen them at puberty.

Our boy's relationship to the opposite sex indicates that he has been only partially successful in accomplishing this task of puberty. Such a failure results form an infantile fixation on some member of the family. it is not normal for an eighteen year old boy to say "a boy doesn't do that when asked if he has ever kissed a girl. We may consider that this strengthens our argument. The boy's statements about his love object deserves our interest. The first girl whom he loved at the age of 13 was the same age as his older sister, her friend and classmate. The two differed little in manner and appearance. His love object is here still the sister, and yet not the sister herself. his present love object has nothing in common with the sister except her work; in appearance she is her opposite in every detail. Does this tell us anything? We know that as the result of repression of the forbidden childish game, everything associated with it is likewise repressed: also that because the love tie to the partner in the game is not really loosened, there is constant danger of its reappearance in reality. The great surge of libido which comes at puberty makes the boy for the first time able to carry out his sexual desires and increases the danger that the sister may become the object of those desires. This danger is lessened if conscious hate blocks the approach to her. It is now possible to understand why the repressed libido had to be changed to hate. The process was accomplished by one of the repressing tendencies which protects the ego. The conscious hate acts as a safety measure and must remain as long as the unconscious erotic tie exists, to prevent its breaking through from the unconscious. It remains a question whether any other tendency was operative to make him give up the sister as sexual object.

Freud has taught us that the surge of libido in puberty is accompanied by a strong wave of repression. This is more powerful in girls than in boys, but in both cases it encounters the early love objects and excludes them as sexual objects. Psychoanalysis says that the incest barrier is erected. The statements of the boy in this case indicate how effective was the repression. We can actually see how this barrier began to raise itself when at 13 he exchanged his sister for the girl similar to her. His present love choice is even more illuminating. The incest barrier has been extended to the type represented by the sister, making the type sexually unapproachable. Yet the youth has not departed from the family. His last love object resembles the youngest sister to whom he is bound by a weaker tie.

Let us formulate our findings in order not to lose perspective. We are discussing an 18-year-old boy who is accused of aggressive behavior at home, especially toward his oldest sister. Our first idea had to be rejected, that the favoritism shown the eldest daughter and the neglect he experienced in childhood led to his dissocial behavior. A memory which he tells of his childhood leads us to believe that this aggression was determined by an unconscious erotic tie to the sister. We were led to this assumption because of the analogous condition to be found in the neurotic, but we found significant facts to confirm it; first, the evidence that the patient's relation to the opposite sex was considerably inhibited, and second the fact that he chose a love object in every way his sister's opposite. I selected this case to present to you because it illustrates many important points in our method of treatment. It shows how deeply we probe for the determining cause of delinquency and how we follow every given clue without waiting for the child to work with us. Our procedure is to set up a picture of the case which will serve to reduce the inevitable element of uncertainty. If you recall that establishing the cause of delinquency was found equivalent to discovering the conditions which had led to latent delinquency, you will understand that we have already fulfilled a part of our purpose. An unconscious erotic tie is one of the psychic conditions that build up a mechanism requiring only a provocation to set it in motion.

Let us now continue our inquiry and consider a remark which the mother made about her son. "He is not a man, just a stupid, stubborn boy." Does this tell us anything? We should compare it with, "He obeys me; he doesn't dare defy me because he knows that I would whip him even though he is 18 years old.... After he has been up to something, he is very obedient and clears up everything around the house nicely." We are inclined to agree that he is not a man; he certainly does not act like one. But does he fit the description of a stupid, stubborn boy? His actions point in another direction. He does the work; about the house usually done by the women. He makes no protest against this; he enjoys it, in fact. His closet is neater than those of his sisters; he stands before the mirror for hours brushing his hair and arranging his tie; he is shy and fearful like a girl. In short, he shows many feminine traits which accord with his appearance. This may be an inherent factor, added to which is the experience of growing up without a father and surrounded only by women. He made no mention of other boys; he spoke only of his sisters and their friends. It often happens that men brought up in a strictly feminine environment develop feminine traits. The fact is unmistakable in this youth. We recognize it not only in his own statements and in what his mother tells us, but we also see it clearly in his whole personality. It is this feminine streak in her son which the mother resents and which causes the boy conflict when he tries to assert his masculinity.

This conflict, which vents itself in outbursts of affect, we may consider the second determinant of his behavior. Are we right in this? Again we must turn to psychoanalysis for deeper insight. We have already learned about identifications, that they are the product of the early attachment of the child to his parents and that if this attachment becomes too strong it will lead to an abnormal development or to delinquency. In order to understand this, we should study the normal psychic development. It will simplify the presentation to discuss the development in the male child only and to assume that of the girl is analogous.

The parents are generally the first persons to enter the sphere of the child's experience, and for this reason the child's first feelings are directed toward them. At first the libidinal strivings of the child are directed equally toward the mother and father; the child love. both equally. In the course of time the feelings for his mother increase, and although he continues to love his father, situations arise which make the father objectionable. Even a three-year-old child can so resent his father's tenderness toward his mother that he would like to get rid of him so that he can have his mother to himself. His feelings for his father now vary; love is at times replaced by rejection. Psychoanalysis describes this as an ambivalent attitude toward the father.

The name chosen by Freud to characterize this unmistakable stage of development has often been misinterpreted. He calls it the Oedipus stage, making reference to the classic myth. You will remember that Oedipus married his mother after killing his father, although neither mother nor son knew of their kinship. Those people who do not wish to understand the psychoanalytic way of thinking raise a cry of indignation at the idea of comparing the relationship between Oedipus and his mother with that of the little boy to his mother. But you who want to understand deserve an explanation. The little boy can no more actually kill his father than he can think of having sexual relations with his mother; his sexual apparatus is too immature. The "Oedipus situation" only signifies the same tendency translated into the emotions of this stage of development, for which the child cannot be held accountable. In psychoanalysis the word "sexual" has come to have a much broader and deeper meaning than was previously the case. As the child's development continues, this negative feeling for his father conflicts with the positive feelings, and is therefore repressed. The real Oedipus situation becomes the Oedipus complex, with all of its repercussions from the unconscious.

If no further disturbances occur, the Oedipus complex is resolved approximately at the beginning of the sixth year. Its resolution marks the time of identification with the parents. The positive Oedipus complex is formed out of the tender relationship to the mother; the negative out of the similar relationship to the father. The first results in a positive attitude toward the mother and a negative attitude toward the father. The second is positive toward the father and negative toward the mother. The positive feelings from both these sources, which in every individual are variously colored by the negative, unite to form a father-and-mother identification. As the growth process continues, these identifications result in a gradual assimilation of the characteristics of the two parents. If the development is not normal-if, for example, the identification with the mother becomes too strong as a result of hereditary or of environmental factors, the boy will acquire female traits and his character will become feminine. The stronger the mother identification becomes, the more the father identification is impaired, and in corresponding measure, all masculine tendencies. The boy grows up deficient in manliness, and his adolescence is prolonged on this account.

This fact had catastrophic importance for the boy in our case. His father died just as he was finishing school at the age of 14. Since he was the oldest child and the only man in the family, he was faced with the task of taking his father's place, Had he been a normally developed boy, he would have been able to do this. But the father identification, which external circumstances forced on him, failed time and again. His mother told us, "He tries to lord it over his sisters, and naturally they won't stand for it. He carries on so and talks so foolishly that the girls laugh at him; this makes him furious and he attacks them like a wild animal." He himself declared with great affect that he was "somebody" and that not only the girls had the say in a household. His inability to act like a man caused him conflict, which he tried to master by excessive brutality. His sisters sensed that he was a cowering woman rather than a forceful man, and made fun of him until he was beside himself with anger. We now have a second explanation for his aggressions. This lack of success in the father identification is clearly the result of his identification with his mother.

But still another conflict disturbed him and helped to determine his behavior. This was the clash of his own socialistic philosophy of life with the strict Catholic ideas of his family. He refused to see any good in their religion, rejected it completely for himself, and yet was too weak to oppose his mother. Instead, he never mentioned the subject, so that his mother was unaware of his real opinion. This resentment also found release in his aggressive behavior. After each outbreak, he gave in and kept on submitting to the mother's authority. In only one thing was his opposition unwavering; he would not become a common laborer. This resistance was reinforced by his determination to show the girl he was fond of that he was worth something. To be a common laborer was to be nothing, and as long as he escaped this destiny, there still remained a chance for him to prove his worth.

We have gone as far in disclosing the determinants of the aggressions of this boy as is necessary' before beginning treatment, We now see that the laziness about which we were consulted is not real laziness. The boy's unfortunate experiences and the opposition of his family have put him in a desperate position. If a change could be brought about in his relationship to his mother and sisters, and if he could find suitable work, it seemed likely that a great improvement would result.

Let us now consider methods of treatment. Above all it seemed important that the boy be spared further experience of failure in the father identification. An easy way to accomplish this was for me to take over the father role in this family for a time. If the boy acknowledged me as the father, he would no longer have to play the part, and one of his conflict situations would be eliminated. With my help he should be able to attain a better relationship with the members of his family. But I would accomplish more if I could bring them into the proper transference relationship to me. The knowledge that I was there, ready to act with father authority if need arose, should change their attitude toward their brother, and the relationship would be improved on both sides. In the same way, the harassed mother would be relieved of anxiety and therefore would be able to adopt a more reasonable attitude toward her son.

This is a superficial description of what takes place in the external situation when the worker steps in to fill the father role in the family. Such external change is all we strive for in the beginning. I did not mention my purpose. The first interview offered possibilities for creating the proper transference. The boy responded at once when he felt he was talking to someone who really understood his misery. The opportunity given her to unburden herself by talking was important in the case of the mother; she left with the feeling of having found someone who could and would help her. She was easily dissuaded from her plan to force the boy out of the house to seek work as a laborer. I was able to arrange that he be given credit for his first year of apprenticeship and go on with learning carpentry. He began work two weeks after our first meeting, and did well. He gave no indication of laziness. We settled the conflict about religion by talking the matter over with his mother. In my presence, the mother promised to allow her son perfect freedom in this respect. After that he no longer joined the family in their social gatherings except when he had the opportunity to meet the girl mentioned earlier.

Doubtless you expect me to tell you the plan that I made for clearing up all his dissocial behavior. But I confess that I am unable to do this, nor am I certain that it would be possible in any case. It has been my practice for years to utilize favorable situations, or, if none exist, to create them; intuition and deliberation serve me alternately, depending on the case. This may seem a very uncertain method, but it may be that ties exist between the unconscious of the analyzed worker and the unconscious of his patient which ensure the accuracy of the work.

It may interest you to hear how the boy reacted during the early part of the treatment. When alone with me, he would scold about his sisters; when we were all together, he played the part of the superior older brother, would look at me with a meaningful nod to see whether I observed how silly the girls were. Peace was restored to the family at the end of a few weeks. The change in atmosphere reacted favorably on each member of the group, although no single member recognized what part he played in bringing this about. The mother's opinion, when asked how things were going, was "much better, he now behaves much more sensibly." The boy attributed the change to the fact that his oldest sister was less disagreeable and that his mother now took his part. I had given the mother some understanding of the boy's conflict, and her changed attitude made the boy feel that she was on his side. For four months I saw the boy two or three times a week, usually not at home. We discussed his aggressive behavior with the result that he came to understand its meaning. At first the outbreaks continued, although they were not so violent as before. They calmed down gradually, and during the last two months of treatment completely disappeared. In this case, the cure was permanent.

CHAPTER NINE
SHAME AND DELINQUENCY

Murray Bilmes

During this century we have gained profound insights into man's mind. Among these are the functions of certain emotions, such as guilt, anxiety, disgust, and shame, in mediating between man's impulsive life and the requirements of civilization. Optimally a person is steered in directions sanctioned by society yet simultaneously establishes a sense of unique being. This affords him both personal satisfactions as well as means and desire to act upon and change the very society that has shaped him. Nevertheless, for many of our youth the world seems to hover between the choice of a long, tedious, uncertain quest for achievement and the plunge into mad but immediate acts of adventure and diversion. The delinquent, in particular, poses a dilemma because of the persistent difficulty, despite the apparently great loss and pain he endures, in coaxing or forcing him into assimilation. Some have sought the causes of this in the inadequacies of our social structure; others in deficiencies of the individual's inner mental structure. Currently, most investigators realize that an adequate answer must somehow fuse these perspectives.

It is in this spirit that I wish to discuss shame and delinquency. My main objective is to detail the enormous burden of shame accompanying male adolescence and relate it to the way our current conventional attitudes toward delinquency give to it a paradoxical face-saving status.

Shame and Guilt

An enormous literature exists on the emotion of guilt, but comparatively little on shame. There is considerable confusion in distinguishing their mental operations. This section will provide a brief review of the salient literature as well as a working definition of shame for this paper.

The early classic psychoanalysts tended to see shame as a reaction formation to exhibitionism.[18,11,8] More recently, the stress has shifted toward viewing shame as a result of tension between the ego and the ego ideal. The importance of ego ideals was emphasized by Freud[12] when he wrote that, "for the ego the formation of an ideal would be the conditioning factor of repression." In the same paper Freud explained the individual's ideal as a "substitute for the lost narcissism of his childhood in which he was his own ideal." Freud described adult pride as constituted of three components: (a)

residues of childish narcissism, (b) object-libido gratification, and ©
fulfillment of the ego ideal. Sandler[23] wrote, "it is possible to suggest. . . that
the affect shame arises when the individual perceives himself (or believes
himself to have been perceived by others) as having failed to live up to ideal
standard which he accepts...". Lynd[17] a sociologist, described shame as, "The
outcome not only of exposing oneself to another person but [also] the
exposure to oneself of parts of the self that one has not recognized and whose
existence one is reluctant to admit." She added later in the same work that,
"there is a particularly deep shame in deceiving other persons into believing
something about oneself that is not true."

The most penetrating study of guilt and shame is the work of Piers and
Singer.[20] These authors state the following as the major properties of shame
which differentiate it from guilt:

1. Shame arises out of a tension between the Ego and the Ego-Ideal,
not between Ego and Super-Ego as in guilt.

2. Whereas guilt is generated whenever a boundary (set by the
Super- Ego) is touched or transgressed, shame occurs when a goal
(presented by the Ego-Ideal) is not being reached. It thus indicates a real "
shortcoming." Guilt anxiety accompanies transgression, shame, failure.

3. The unconscious, irrational threat implied in shame anxiety is
abandonment and not mutilation (castration) as in guilt.

4. The Law of Talion does not obtain in the development of shame,
as it generally does in guilt.

Guilt, then, is seen as the sense of having done something wrong, shame
the sense of having failed to live up to one's desired image. This in turn
refers to differing purposes of the superego and the ego ideal, a distinction
succinctly stated by Sandler [23] as, "The superego sets boundaries for the ego,
the ego ideal goals" and by A. Reich[22] as, "The ego ideal expresses what one
desires to be, the superego what one ought to be".

It is a unique aspect of human mentality for a set of ideals to develop
gradually. Their consistency and inner lack of contradiction plus the ability
to live up to or move in the direction of fusing what Rado[21] calls the tested
sense of self with those images of a desired self constitute a major part of a
person's sense of well-being-his sense of having an identity and a vantage
point from which to perceive and relate himself to the world. The
confirmation of others is also important for the quality this experience has.
In addition, everyone clears, in part, with the disharmony between the self as
one sees it and the self as one ideally wants to see it by trying to appear to

have the missing qualities. We might call this the assumed self. The potential danger of the disparity between these aspects of self being exposed constitutes the potential for shame anxiety and it is in this sense that shame is used in this paper. Shame when present may, like guilt, be unconscious or it may break out in raw form or in one of its derivatives like embarrassment, timidity, humiliation, inferiority, inadequacy, and so on. It is my belief that a great part of the adolescent's struggle is his effort to knit these various divisions within his psyche. Later in life other processes are used to deal with residual unknit factors, such as modification of the ideals in the direction of diminishing or diffusing them, but in adolescence their tensions are at their most acute and powerful point of interplay.

Effects of Shame

The unrelenting and pervasive persistence of this emotion has been grippingly portrayed by Joseph Conrad in his novel, *Lord Jim*. After a crushing shame incident, in which Jim, a ship's officer, abandons a seemingly sinking ship with the passengers still on board, Jim spends the remainder of his life restlessly drifting, seeking, and, ultimately, finding a way to redeem himself. It is important to differentiate this type of redemption, resulting from shame, from the type due to guilt. Guilt can be expiated through penance, atonement, self-punishment, good works, but shame-the exposed rent in one's image-can only be overcome through a change in this image. Significantly this can even be done to some extent without real inner change. Success in merely giving a certain appearance to others can itself diminish shame.

This touches on a vital issue. What does a person do to get rid of the sense of shame? One obvious technique is concealment and hiding. In the Adam and Eve myth the immediate consequence of eating of the forbidden fruit is the experience of shame, first before each other, then before God. In both instances they clear with their shame by concealment. Erikson[7] has stated that "shame is early expressed in an impulse to bury one's face, or to sink, right then and there, into the ground."

A second technique is to try to be accepted by one's group in order to attain, one might say, a state of grace and forgiveness. This is frequently done through conformity and, while guilt mechanisms may lead to similar behavior, social conformity resulting from shame is essentially one of identification, whereas social conformity prompted by guilt is essentially one of submission.

A third major way to eliminate shame is through seeking special kinds of achievements, often called heroic, which lead to image enhancement, restored pride and ultimately, as the Japanese expression puts it, the saving of face.

These last points, all dealing with means of shame riddance, are basic to my attempt to explain why the experience of shame in adolescence may lead to the adoption of a delinquent way of life.

In an earlier paper[3] I reported that among the adolescents I studied shame was more powerful than guilt. By that I meant to emphasize two things in particular: (1) It is easier to motivate an adolescent or to spur him into action through an appeal to his sense of shame than to his guilt. In other words, telling him not to do something because it is wrong will often have a negligible effect while saying, for instance, that he is a coward (or, as it would be put on the street, that he is "chicken," or "yellow," or a "sissy," or "soft") if he does not do something will almost always produce a very appreciable effect. (2) That admitting to guilt is for many adolescents a sign of weakness, of unmanliness, a violation of the basic code of the streets-being hard-and the shame of such admission plays a significant role in masking the usual manifestations of guilt or conscience.

The reasons for this can be reduced to what is perhaps an over-simplification (though not an inaccurate one) by stating that *adolescent culture is intrinsically a shame culture*.

The major problems of the adolescent include achievement, pride, masculine identity, passivity, sexual success, independence, and attaining a position of respect. To fail in any of these is a loss of face and a humiliation. The soft underbelly of all these problems is the experience of shame.

Shame and Adolescence

Certain social factors, unique to our time, make the adolescent especially vulnerable to shame. There is, for example, the problem of achievement. Achievement has always been valued but perhaps never as in our age, when it is actually considered shameful to stand still and not keep advancing oneself. Never have achievement and education been as intimately linked as they now are. Today a lack of formal education almost certainly dooms a man to a life of ignominy. The range of opportunity for unskilled labor, let alone the dignity attached to it, has shrunk astonishingly. As automation continues to envelop our society, the place for the uneducated seems certain to vanish. We can see this in such diverse occupations, as construction, running an elevator, agriculture, or soldiering. Everywhere the prospect for the uneducated or relatively uneducated is the same-a morass of futility, failure, and insignificance. It is certain that one of the major problems for our society is and will become even more so, the question of what to with that portion of our population whose image of itself is loaded with a sense of failure and self- derogation.

Another-special problem of our society is its unusual attempt to synthesize unbounded prosperity and unbounded freedom of rights. With so much available, it is hard to live with oneself if only a small part of the wealth and success is possessed. In former times, traditional institutions, such as religion or the economic structure of society itself, as in feudalism, made it possible for a person to live with relatively little and still possess a sense of dignity. He could explain to himself why he did not have more. But today what can be told to a man who sees others-and with the mass media of TV, movies and magazines, the tremendous pressure of advertisement, he is bound to see others-having so much more? His philosophy of the democratic life tells him that he has the same rights, the same opportunities as others, and yet the consequences are so different. It is no use telling him he is better off than a wealthy man from a previous century who did not have even toilet facilities in his apartment. The fact is that psychologically he is not better off. Self-judgment is partly based on the differential between oneself and others and the explanations used to account for this differential. Today the man who has less is more likely to conclude he is a failure. Having less becomes a blow to pride, a source of shame. Moreover, the inexhaustibility of products and illusory fulfillment of needs, both real and artificial, helps create an awesome state of anomie, for the sense of "enough" loses all meaning. Let me quote Durkheim[6] to you on this:

". .. how is one to determine exactly the amount of well-being of comfort, of luxury, to which a human being can legitimately aspire? If neither the organic nor the psychological constitution of man is anything to be found which sets a boundary to such propensities.... Therefore, insofar as they depend upon the individual alone, these desires are boundless. In itself, disregarding all external forces which control it, our capacity for feeling is a bottomless abyss which nothing could fill.

But then, if no external force limits our feeling, it can be by itself nothing but a source of pain. For unlimited desires are insatiable by definition, and it is not without reason that insatiability is regarded as a sign of morbidity...

To the extent that appetites are not curbed automatically by physiological mechanisms, they cannot be halted except by a limitation which they themselves recognize as just.... Only society ... is in a position to play this restraining role....

...When society is disturbed or disorganized, whether by a painful crisis or by a fortunate but too sudden turn of events, it is incapable of exercising this influence upon the individual....

If the disturbance originates in an abrupt increase in power and wealth . . .people no longer feel sure about what is possible and what is not....The richer prize offered to them stimulates them, makes them more exacting, more impatient of every rule, just at the time when traditional rules have lost their authority. The state of rulelessness or anomie is further heightened by the fact that human desires are less disciplined at the very moment when they would need a stronger discipline....

From top to bottom of the social scale, violent but indefinite and unfocused desires are aroused. Reality seems worthless compared with what these fevered imaginations conceive to be possible; thus people abandon reality, only to abandon the possible when it in turn becomes real. They thirst for novelty, for unknown delights, for nameless sensations, which nevertheless lose all their zest as soon as they are experienced".

These words are almost prophetic for our age with its tremendous impact on our youth. The emotional crisis so engendered cannot, of course, be reduced to any one single item. Where others perhaps would stress the problems of the formation of a sense of self, or of identity, I wish to add the emphasis on the role of the concomitant sense of shame-a shame compounded of futility, failure, and the diminution of a base of standards on which to build a sense of pride.

Among discriminated minority groups still other factors contribute to this condition. It has been pointed out[5,16] that one of the most vicious aspects of discrimination is that the discriminated person becomes ashamed of himself and sees himself through the eyes of the prejudice carriers. This often extends beyond oneself to include one's parents and family roots. In this way, the feeling of family solidarity, a source of one of the basic restraining forces integrating a person into society, is fragmented and repudiated. Many analysts, including Anna Freud in a particularly stimulating paper[10] on adolescence, have convincingly demonstrated how acutely infantile patterns of dependency become reactivated in adolescence. It is at this time that the adolescent is urged in our society to become emotionally independent of his parents. Up to a point this is helpful, even necessary, in aiding the adolescent grow into a self-sufficient individual. But there is also danger in too sharply prohibiting dependency needs. Any closeness at all to parents may become associated with a humiliating infantilism, and needs that could become sources of tenderness and warmth in human relations may be radically denigrated, helping to provide what Suttie[25] so aptly called a "tenderness taboo." Among many delinquents this has gotten translated into the sense that emotions like compassion, considerateness, and love are stigmata of weakness and effeminacy, and therefore shameful.*

Moreover, the massive movement of our population to urban ways of life, the incredibly large numbers of people met everyday have helped create a dehumanizing attitude toward people. City life *requires* the development of a dehumanizing attitude. Without it one could not adapt to a structure by which people are often experienced only as objects, as things that crowd one's space and must be emotionally neutralized. This attitude affects the adolescent in two major ways. On the one hand he is himself the recipient of such regard from others and his sense of self-worth is thereby demeaned and frustrated. At the same time, in viewing others, it helps foment the feeling that stealing from them, mugging them, sometimes even murdering them, is an impersonal act as devoid of human sentiment as kicking a stone. The statistics of war casualties we read and hear about every day-generally stated with considerably more matter of-factness than the temperature reading-is an illustration of this attitude.

To these problems must be added the many others faced by adolescents in our culture. To list just a few-there is the tremendous competition for placement in school, in attaining excellence in athletics, and in being popular; there is the curious blend of puritanism, lasciviousness, and pleasure-seeking, of the contradiction in teaching Judaeo-Christian ethics with simultaneous propensity to ruthless pursuit of personal goals of success and power.

These facets of contemporary life create in many adolescents a massive need to overcome an inner sense of inferiority, insignificance, damaged self-esteem, and pride. There is a constant and painful threat to their ego ideal and hence constant vulnerability to exposure and shame.

Whereas some societies have recognized through rites of passage and puberty rituals the need to formally help the individual gain a stable sense of self, our present civilization has so far been unable to find ways to doing this. Accordingly, other activities have preempted this purpose. A recent

---

* Anna Freud makes the interesting point that while it is generally accepted that a strong fixation to mother makes adolescence difficult, it is essential for the adolescent to have a stable mother figure image in order to adequately transfer feelings to new objects.

publication⁴ pointed out the many congruences between gang habits and primitive puberty rites. An obvious illustration, for example, is the initiation procedures found in both. Whereas the initiation rite in primitive society helps the youth become identified with the larger society, gang initiation furthers the separateness of the adolescent from his adult society. Thus, gangs are relatively unstable and cast adrift in the world, their tensions and contained emotions often spilling over into violence thrill-seeking, and a vague search of adventure. Without real roots, the true source of experience is absent. Pleasure-seeking seems often to be only a substitute for this inability to experience.

Other factors that have been stressed as important for understanding the adolescent are often, when examined more carefully, aspects of shame; for example, the presence of inferiority feelings. What is painful about inferiority feelings, however, is the release of shameful exposure in inadequately matching up to some ideal image for oneself. Superiority of another yields pain only because it makes us feel inadequate and failing in some respect. The fear of failure, as Karen Horney saw,¹⁴ "is in part an expression of the fear of being humiliated."

It is, as I mentioned earlier, the hallmark of man to develop ideals and an image he wishes to live up to, to identify with, and present as his spiritual face to the outside; but it is also true that life-even in the most successful-imposes severe compromises on these strivings; the most humbling force in life is life itself.

All of us, as we get older, protect ourselves from having to be disturbed by our shortcomings by shrinking our expectations and our ego ideal, or shifting them onto other things and people.

For example, we turn the other into a kind of myth-he's a "genius," or "a hero," "in a class by himself"-in order not to bring ourselves into comparison with him. The adolescent also does this. He will, for example, elevate certain members of his group into leadership status. His pride then avoids the shame of an unfavorable comparison, and also he can then actually build his pride by participating in the glory or patronage of the leader. The adolescent is, and should be, filled with the need to follow his ego's own rising star. By the same token, he is all the more vulnerable to having his aspirations tarnished.

Shame and Delinquency

Adolescents build their pride and avoid being ashamed of themselves through identification with heroic figures or through the creation of a heroic role for themselves. When stymied, this effort becomes contaminated, as Alexander[2] pointed out, with increased aggressiveness, with fantasying oneself to be superior, or with depreciative competition. For, as Erikson said: "too much shaming does not result in a sense of propriety but in a secret determination to try to get away with things when unseen, if, indeed, it does not result in shamelessness."

Defending by retreat and hiding is difficult because it is a defense that engenders even more shame. This is because our societal values applaud extroverted, demonstrable patterns of life. Not only patterns of retreat but any kind of seriousness, introversion, artistic and intellectual pursuit can mark one for the brand of sissy. The cartoon of the boy with the violin case being jeered at by his adolescent acquaintances is a familiar stereotype.

Often, therefore, as Erikson put it, "he who is ashamed would like to force the world not to look at him, not to notice his exposure. *He would like to destroy the eyes of the world*" (italics mine).

It is striking that criminal and delinquent activities provide a way of doing just this, of obliterating that segment of reality which, if emotionally accepted, means accepting the shame.

> A patient of mine, placed in boarding school, was found masturbating by one of the supervisors and then made an example of to the school. The result, naturally, was that he felt totally humiliated and became the butt of everyone's ridicule. A month after this incident he began an extensive series of thefts from the other boys as well as the school.

If he had continued to respect the reality of the world of the boarding school, it would have meant continuing to respect its values and its judgment of him- a dirty masturbator. With his thefts he was expressing his rage at this world, denying its authority and hold over him and simultaneously building a new image of himself (a clever thief, a man who took what he wanted, not a weak, goody-goody like the others).

In fact, the two most common aspects of contemporary delinquency, violence and drug addiction, are alternate ways of destroying reality. In the one case it is done quite literally and physically while in the other it is done by destroying the ability' within oneself to be affected by it. In addition, these two means of destroying reality actually help create a new kind of reality and a new status with respect to it. To demand of the delinquent, then, that he admit - his wrongs, reform his ways, is to ask of him precisely that which would shatter his major source of status and pride, is to ask him to openly avow his inadequacy and fully face his humiliation and shame. Let me emphasize this by putting it another way: for the delinquent, the problem of becoming a decent, law abiding citizen is not that he would feel guilty in not doing this, but rather that he would feel *declasse*, reduced to a mediocrity and a nonentity, in doing it.

Fenichel[*] noted that ambition is a fight against shame. An article by Harry Slochower[24] carried this point further by arguing that "one of the motivations for delinquent behavior is a desire to assume a heroic role" and that the delinquent way of life provides such a heroic role. Perhaps significant in this connection is Churchill's description of Hitler, as that "monstrous product of past wrongs and shame."

Many will recoil from this idea out of the feeling that delinquency is reprehensible, criminal, wicked, vicious. So it is, but this misses the point. An evil thing can attain heroic proportions. The tremendous fear of the populace, the awesome fascination with delinquency, so cleverly exploited by the mass media in order to sell their products, not infrequently even found among workers with delinquents who wind up emulating their style of dress and speech, is pathetic testimony of this. Lucifer's famous line in Milton's *Paradise Lost* epitomizes this mood: "Better to reign in hell than serve in heaven."

One may identify with what is evil but never with what is shameful. Evil figures exercise notorious fascination and power of attraction. *Evil is compatible with identification, shame is not!* Voltaire once said, "I have never made but one prayer to God, a very short one: 'O Lord, make my enemies ridiculous,' " and, as Robert White[27] pointed out, "the one invariant affect [in identification] is admiration of the model."

We have now arrived at the paradox in dealing with delinquency. The more we publicize it, the more we condemn it, the more we fear it, the more we associate it with evil-the more dramatic and heroic a model it becomes for certain of our youth. We create a highly idealized and desirable image.

Therapy of the Delinquent

In dealing with the problem of forest fires, there must be techniques for dealing with specific fires as well as techniques and plans for general forest management. Treating the delinquent, in this sense, is no different. The individual has to be treated, but a broader approach at the community level is also necessary. This section will discuss treatment of the individual; the next section will discuss proposals at the community level.

The task of treating the delinquent-and generally this is primarily taken to mean the elimination of delinquent behavior rather than deep-seated characterological alteration as sought by traditional psychoanalysis-must pay more attention to the handling of shame and its derivatives. I believe that this also holds true for the treatment of related conditions, such as narcotic addiction and alcoholism.

As Piers pointed out: "It is at times of great importance for the general understanding of the case as well as for the immediate interpretative task which one of the two anxiety forms (that is, guilt anxiety and shame anxiety) one has to deal with, or whether one is concealing the other."

> Piers described a patient who insisted on paying at the end of each session because he couldn't trust himself to otherwise remember. The therapy went downhill when Piers attempted to discuss the patient's guilt feeling about depriving him of his fee. Only later did he realize that the patient experienced therapy as shameful and his need to pay at the each session was a way of saving face by putting the therapist in his place as a hired hand....The shame-driven patient's unconscious experienced my gesture of trust and encouragement as an additional humiliation which widened the gulf between his (imagined) inferiority and my (projected) superiority. Similarly the therapeutic effort to get a patient to experience and express his hostilities might be decisive in certain cases of guilt-repressed aggressiveness. But to concentrate on the hostilities of the shame-driven will miss the point of his main problem. It might play in with his defense of overcompensation, or it might help to conceal the shame behind the guilt.... it does not follow at all that a pathological condition with the nuclear problem of shame will yield to therapy easier than one of guilt. Rather the opposite is true.... Our culture strongly emphasizes comparing and competing-causative to shame tension, and on the other hand, puts a premium on compensatory activity. This makes extremely difficult the therapeutic task of delimiting adaptive techniques from neurotic acting out.

It is helpful to view the delinquent's behavior as a means of acting his inner fantasies out on the real world and its objects in much the same manner as a child acts its fantasies out on play material provided it. Moreover, the delinquent is seeking to project an image through this behavior, which he then seeks to believe in, or identify himself with, as being his true self. Often the best way of cutting through this behavior is to expose the shame elements beneath it.

> A young adolescent patient of mine had been sparking a group that burglarized stores and apartments in a rural area. He was somewhat afraid of being caught when he read local newspaper accounts of the thefts but mostly gained a tremendous sense of heightened self- esteem through them. One evening, at a bowling alley, another kid, derisively called "shrimp" by his acquaintances, came in and showed the others some articles he had

stolen from a store that afternoon. My patient felt disgusted and humiliated that he had, for several months, been doing exactly what this "shrimp" had done. He forthwith gave up the burglarizing, feeling it was now beneath him. Theft had lost status for him in precisely the same way that it was an attempt to earn it for the "shrimp."

Another youngster, constantly stressing how ashamed he was of his father, because of the latter's immigrant status, continual inability to earn much of a living, and general timidity before others, had begun experimenting with "pot," become a behavioral problem at school because of his bullying, and had just finished constructing a zip gun. He claimed he had to do this in order to keep up with and earn the respect of the others. One day he told me how his father had come to leave his native country. He had refused to salute Hitler during a street parade, been arrested, placed in a concentration camp, then escaped and eventually made his way to America. When I contrasted the courage of his father in daring to oppose others, even at terrible risk to himself, with what I called in this boy his cowardice in standing up against his own crowd, he became embarrassed. This incident, often referred to by me, was a major source of leverage which eventually led to this boy's renouncing his delinquent patterns. I do not think that trying to activate latent guilt feelings would have been as helpful.

Certain group organizations, like AA and Synanon, while carefully eschewing outright moral condemnation for the addict, actually employ a variety of shaming and hazing techniques to force the changes they seek. One phase of this in Synanon is called "attack therapy," sometimes going to the point of shaving the delinquent's head and then verbally abusing him while he stands bald-headed in front of them. Simultaneously, these organizations provide a new status and prestige to those who successfully kick their habit and stay clean.

In the psychotherapy of the delinquent I do not think it is enough merely to expose the elements of shame; it is essential to explore the many ways in which the delinquent patterns serve to provide a means of overcoming the shame anxiety and, where possible, to make the continuance of the delinquency itself a source of shame rather than of bogus heroism. Most important is also the search for new patterns of pride, self-esteem, and self-respect. More attention ought to be given to the quality of courage-a very real emotional problem for the adolescent. Hemingway is reported to have once said to a group of psychoanalysts, "You fellows know a lot about fear but you don't know anything about courage." Most analysts, sitting in their offices, successful in their careers, generally "pillars of society," vastly removed from the world of physical challenge as they deftly explore the power of verbal exchange, often do not grasp the real terror for the adolescent of cowardice and his imperative need to demonstrate courage in physical terms. In the adolescent, man's most primitive needs, the aggressive and sexual, are confronted with their moment of truth. It is essential that therapy be concerned with helping the adolescent face these issues with strength, not shame.

I have found it helpful, in attempting to do this, to focus on the adolescent's daydream. Of the case histories found in the current literature, while many cite dreams and their analyses, they rarely discuss daydreams. Yet, in adolescence, daydreams are a particularly rich source for tracing how the individual is trying to cope with his omnipotent and narcissistic frustrations and blows to his self-esteem. Masturbatory fantasies, for example, are common and obviously among those most powerfully linked to feelings of shame. Sometimes such a fantasy is elaborated in more disguised ways.

> One adolescent patient, a fire setter, who felt puny and physically inferior to other boys, used to repetitively daydream of hitting home-runs. In his fantasy he would contemplate with rapture the flight of the ball as it soared over the outfield, over the bleachers, and, finally, out over the ball park. He recalled how when he was a little boy, he would stand at the curb, urinate into the street, and watch the trajectory of his urine.

A common pattern in the delinquent is the promotion of aggressiveness as a mask for his passive-dependent feelings which, in turn, he is deeply ashamed of. It is important in the individual therapy of the delinquent to elicit these underlying dependency strivings and to undo the shame connected with them.

> An adolescent I treated had spent years as the sissy of the block. He was taunted, punched, and patronizingly tolerated. He then adopted a technique of using his weaknesses to draw laughs out of the others. The purpose seemed to be that of warding off ridicule by fronting as the court jester of his street. Secretly he nursed a deep resentment that inevitably came out through a variety of invidious, devious practices. He was also afraid of girls. As he reached late adolescence he gradually developed an unmistakably paranoid cast. He eyed everyone with suspicion, secretly fancied himself, when alone in his room, as an SS officer who carried out barbaric, sadistic tortures upon innumerable persons under his control. He bought boots that he wore constantly, carried a switchblade, and became a chronic user of marijuana, a "pothead." The boy was filled with fears of becoming a homosexual and, if you wish, of castration anxiety. His paranoid-like overlay may seem like confirmation of Freud's hypothesis of the connecting link between paranoia and homosexuality and perhaps it is, but more to the point, in my opinion, is not the fear of homosexuality as such, but the fear of the shame it implied. As we began to discuss this feeling, he eventually described his desire to dig a hole "500 feet deep"

to hide himself in. Finding the courage to face these thoughts and tell them
to me in itself heightened his self-respect. The "homosexuality" he spoke
of mostly had to do with his passivity and sense of inferiority; the SS
fantasies were misguided gropings at compensation.

Nyswander[9] has clearly delineated the same dynamics in the drug
addicts she worked with:

> Once their thin layer of bravado is gone, their profound feelings of
> inadequacy are revealed, [a] complete lack of self-confidence in their
> ability to compete successfully with other men in society.... After they
> have discussed their feelings of inadequacy to cope with the outside
> world, they invariably quickly turn to their successes in the drug addict
> world: the important people they know, their ability to obtain drugs at any
> time, and their wide connections with peddlers. It is as if their self-
> importance in the world of drug addicts must be built up to
> counterbalance their failure in the outside world....
>
> On casual observance the drug addict does not reveal his low self-
> esteem but may instead appear cocky and boastful. His life is seen as a
> perpetual denial that he has any such low opinion of himself....
>
> His [the drug addict's] need for success makes him withdraw from all
> activities, for he can't take the chance that he might fail in any of them. .
> . . He shuns any situation which he cannot control and in which he may be
> exposed in an unfavorable light. Appearing to have no interest in what he
> is doing is a face-saving device, in case he should fail it would seem that
> he couldn't care less....
>
> As a substitute he finds a group with a different set of values, one
> which respects daring and bravado, one in which he can control the
> outcome of his behavior. To win over this group he is willing to be the
> sacrificial lamb; he volunteers to accept any dare made to the group, and
> in a short time he can exhibit himself in the role of a "big shot"....
>
> . . . as long as [drugs] . . . are forbidden, the addict will meet the
> challenge of defying the law to get them. Acquiring the forbidden has
> given the addict another chance to achieve a feeling of superiority over
> others, and by outwitting the authorities he can look on himself as their
> superior in intelligence and resourcefulness.

Thomas French[9] finds this to hold true in the treatment of the alcoholic as
well:

> The aggressive protest of an alcoholic against his dependent
> cravings may take such disturbing forms that we are tempted to reject
> him as a hopeless case. If we overcome our irritation, however, and
> look for the rationale behind this disturbing behavior, we discover that
> this aggressive protest is only an excessive... manifestation of the
> very incenltive that must be utilized in helping him learn to play a

more independent role. At first *he is so ashamed* of his intense dependent cravings that he must use all his aggressive energy in attempts to deny them (italics mine).

It is significant that even where feelings of guilt appear to be shockingly absent, shame emotions may not. In March of 1964, the country was stunned by the murder in Queens, New York, of Kitty Genovese. She was stalked through the street and to the hallway of an apartment building, stabbed, killed, then sexually molested. Some 35 people were reported to have witnessed some aspect of this murder without any of them calling the police. The murderer, William Mosey, insisted he felt no remorse over the deed. When police led him by a battery of cameramen, however, he said: "I have a father out there. I also have a wife, and this is a pretty *shameful thing.* Would it be all right with you people if I covered up my face?"

Especially critical in the treatment of the delinquent is the struggle to elicit feelings of affection, confidence, and love. For ultimately, the capacity to feel strength in these emotions is the greatest safeguard against the hardness that makes possible the unfeeling violence against what is felt as an impersonal world, filled with impersonal people. Perhaps the single most crucial quality needed by someone working with delinquents is the ability to stimulate in the youth a desire to affectionately emulate and identify with him. Nevertheless, as Aichhorn[1] has pointed out, the time when the delinquent youth begins to feel affection for his therapist is a delicate time. For an unintended rejection will turn the affection back into hate. The reason for this is probably the shame of having made a fool of oneself (in the delinquent's eyes) by permitting oneself to feel affection (which is often taken to be synonymous with showing it) in vain. An attitude of unremitting hardness offers a special protection against exposure to this type of humiliation and is therefore one of the reasons that the hard-boiled exterior of many delinquents is so difficult to penetrate. In the same vein Lewis Hill[b] noted that ". .. It has seemed to me that feelings of dependence, of a need to be loved, or passivity and helplessness . . . and even feelings of affection can seem so intolerable to certain patients that they prefer to show themselves. as ill- tempered and defiant, quarrelsome or threatening."

Sometimes society provides vicious outlets for such people, like the SS of which my patient fantasied himself a member, or the Ku Klux Klan in our own society. In fact, a number of years ago Wertham[26] stirred up considerable controversy by arguing that comics and TV were to blame for stimulating acts of violence in impressionable youngsters. Aside from how much or little, one accepted his conclusions, it helped focus on the question of what the community, and the mass media at its disposal, can do to avert delinquent acts.

The Community Approach to Delinquency

William James[15] once discussed the need to find a "moral equivalent of war." I believe that today he would urge us to seek a moral equivalent of delinquency. As James puts it:

> ... men at large still live as they always have lived, under a pain-and-fear economy- for those of us who live in an ease-economy are but an island in the stormy ocean-and the whole atmosphere of present day utopian literature tastes mawkish and dishwatery to people who still keep a sense for life's more bitter flavours. It suggests, in truth, ubiquitous inferiority. Inferiority is always with us, and merciless scorn of it is the keynote of the military temper... The best thing about our inferiors today is that they are as though asnails, and physically and morally almost as insensitive. Utopianism would see them soft and squeamish, while militarism would keep their callousness, but transfigure it into a meritorious characteristic, needed by the service and redeemed by that from the suspicion of inferiority. No collectivity is like an army for nourishing such pride; but it has to be confessed that the only sentiment which the image of pacific cosmopolitan industrialism is capable of arousing . . . is shame at the idea of belonging to such a collectivity. [James then goes to argue that there should be a conscription of the whole youthful population to form for a certain number of years an army enlisted against nature, where a manly "blood tax" would be enacted by working the youth in mines, fishing fleets, tunnel making, foundries and the frames of skyscrapers. In this manner, "we could get toughness without callousness."]

> So far [James continues] war has been the only force that can discipline a whole community, and until an equivalent discipline is organized, I believe that war must have its way. But I have no serious doubts that the ordinary prides and shames of social man .. . are capable of organizing such a moral equivalent. . . it is but a question of time, of skillful propagandism, and of opinion-making men seizing historic opportunities.

Can we do this with delinquency? Competitive sports, of course, provide one way. These should continue to be greatly encouraged and financially supported by our communities. And the range of activities should be as broad as possible so as to bring in as many of our youth as possible-the range should go from football to chess. What James spoke about, was, in part, brilliantly achieved by the late President Kennedy through the Peace Corps. The same elements- adventure, thrills, courage, prestige-that so often promote delinquency were here utilized constructively. Social planners should give more attention to the creation of other programs serving the same purpose. Otherwise, the mere alleviation of poverty and slums, while certainly of great importance, will not succeed in building self-respect and avoiding the shame of self. The rise in delinquency among our wealthy youngsters amply demonstrates this.

The other major change that the community could undertake is to take the glamour out of delinquency. Ideally we should strive to reach a point where delinquent acts, instead of helping relieve shame, increase it. Perhaps this is one reason why many addicts and delinquents go through the process called "maturing out" in which they seem to outgrow their youthful behavior. While stealing from the "Five-and-Ten" may seem heroic to a sixteen-year-old it must, in the eyes of the same person at the age of thirty-five, appear somewhat humiliating. While the sixteen-year old can boast of such a feat to others and gain status, it would be absurd for the same person to do so at thirty-five.

If we could prevail upon the representatives of the mass media, editors, reporters, and news commentators on radio and TV, I would make this suggestion: Every time an act of delinquency of whatever type is reported, avoid calling it "bad," "evil," "wicked," "monstrous," and other words of this type, because they only make the delinquent feel he has done something big and important. Instead use words like "cowardly," "silly," "infantile," "yellow"-that is, write up or tell the incidents in a way likely to make the act appear humiliating to its perpetrator. As I have stated before, this is the most effective way of rendering a role unsuitable for identification-by making it shameful and ridiculous. Its corollary, I repeat, is that making a role evil enhances its identification value.

In the 1930's there was the popular stereotype of the "mad" scientist. This image was seemingly highly effective in deterring large numbers of youth from entering this field. When the government realized its need to encourage youth to enter the sciences, it very wisely and successfully waged a mass propaganda campaign designed to glamorize the sciences. What I am suggesting, with respect to delinquency, is that our society move exactly the opposite way.

Finally, I think more thought ought to be given to the use of shame as a deterrent in the fields of education and in the legal use of punishments. Traditionally, punishments were of a shame as well as the guilt type. Instead of the "eye for an eye" philosophy or its derivatives, x years for burglary, both based on the notion that one "pays" for one's crime and is then quits with society and inner conscience, other punishments-like the scarlet letter or public exposure and ridicule in the pillory were used because they *shamed* the offender. I am not arguing for the return of these specific techniques, only for a re-examination of the principle underlying them.

There is of course the danger that too much shame will drive the delinquent even further into a need for renewed delinquencies. Our guilt punishment system, however, has not been notable for its success in reducing recidivism. The judicious use of shame threats as punishment may be a powerful deterrent, directed not only against the delinquent but also against his family. Furthermore, instead of shaming the delinquent it is possible to "punish" him in the opposite direction-to press him into a conscription-a kind of updated Foreign Legion, whose duties and assignments require a high degree of daring and adventure. This daring and adventure, of course, would be in the service of objectives having social utility and would be another aspect of the "moral equivalent of delinquency," mentioned earlier, except in this instance it would be imposed as a punishment on the individual for the delinquent acts he committed.

SUMMARY

The theme of this paper has been the significance of the function of shame in understanding delinquent behavior. Adolescent culture is largely a shame culture. The many influences on the adolescent, making him especially vulnerable to shame emotions, impel him to seek ways of compensation. The most prevalent form of this is an attempt to forge a heroic self image. Aspects of the delinquent role, though opposed by dictates of conscience, nevertheless exert great allure because of their many face saving and ego enhancing possibilities.

In the psychotherapy of the delinquent, particular attention should be given to the presence of shame and the defenses erected against it. Often, for example, the mistake is made of dealing with reported acts and fantasies of violence as if the crux of the matter resided in eliciting feelings of guilt and conscience or in tracing out the roots of the feelings of hate and rage. The presence of underlying acts and fantasies related to passivity, weakness, despondency, and so on-of which the delinquent is deeply ashamed, is overlooked. Consequently, the way in which the delinquent act is a means of masking the shame is also missed. Shame needs to be carefully differentiated from guilt. In general, guilt pertains to the sense of having done something wrong and shame to the sense of failing to live up to one's desired self image. It also appears that while it is possible to desire to identify with an "evil" image this is never the case with a shameful image.

There is a general impression nowadays that the work of the therapist in the consulting room is unrelated to the problems of the community at large. This paper endeavors to demonstrate that an understanding of the role of shame in delinquent behavior also leads to suggestions of how to deal with this problem at the community level.

REFERENCES

1. Aichhorn, A., *Wayward Youth* (New York: Meridian Books, 1955).
2. Alexander, F., "Remarks About The Relation of Inferiority Feelings to Guilt Feelings," *Int. J. Psychoanal*, (1938), 41.
3. Bilmes, M., "The Delinquent's Escape From Conscience", *Am. J. Psychother.* 19 (1965), 633. '
4. Bloch, H., and Niederhoffer, A., *The Gang* (New York: Philosophical Library, 1958).
5. Clark, K., and Clark, K., "Racial Identification and Preference in Negro Children," in *Readings In Social Psychology*, eds. T. M. Newcomb and E. L. Hartley (New York: Henry Holt, 1947).
6. Durkheim, E., "Anomie," in *Images of Man*, ed. C. W.Mills (New York: George Braziller, 1960).
7. Erikson, E., "Identity and The Life Cycle," in *Psychological Issues* (New York Int. Univ. Press, 1959).
8. Fenichel, O., *The Psychoanalytic Theory of Neurosis* (New York: W. W. Norton, 1945).
9. French, I., "The Transference Phenomenon," in *Psychoanalytic Therapy*, eds. F. Alexander and T. French (New York: Ronald Press, 1946). Ch. 5.
10. Freud, A,. "Adolescence," in *The Psychoanalytic Study of the Child*, Vol. 13 (New York: Int. Univ. Press, 1958), pp. 255-278.
11. Freud,S., "Three Essays on Sexuality" in *Standard Edition*, Vol. 7 (London: Hogarth Press, 1953),
12. -, "On Narcissism," in *Collected Papers*, Vol. 4 (London: Hogarth Press, 1948).
13. Hill, L., "The Use of Hostility as a Defence," *Psychoanal. Quart.*, 7 (1938), 254.
14. Horney, K., *The Neurotic Personality of Our Time* (New York: W.W.Norton, 1937).
15. James, W., "The Moral Equivalent of War," in *William James*, ed. M.

Knight (London: Penguin Books, 1950).

16. Kardiner, A., *The Mark of Oppression* (New York: W. W. Norton, 1951).

17. Lynd, H., *On Shame and The Search For Identity* (New York: Harcourt, Brace, 1958).

18. Nunberg, H, *Principles of Psychoanalysis* (New York: Int. Univ. Press, 1955).

19. Nyswander, M., *The Drug Addict as a Patient* (New York: Grune & Stratton, 1956).

20. Piers, G., and Singer, M., *Shame and Guilt* (Springfield, 111.: C. C Thomas,

21. Rado, S., *Psychoanalysis of Behavior.* (New York: Grune & Stratton, 1956).

22. Reich, A., "Early Identification as Archaic Elements in the Superego," *J. Amer. Psychoanal. Ass.*, 2 (1954), 84.

23. Sandler, J., Holder A., and Meers, D., "The Ego Ideal and The Ideal Self," in *The Psychoanalytic Study of the Child*, Vol. 18 (New York: Int. Univ. Press 1963).

24. Slochower, H., "The Juvenile Delinquent and the Mythic Hero," *Dissent* (Summer 1961), 413.

25. Suttie, I., *Origins of Love and Hate* (London: Kegan Paul, 1935).

26. Wertham, F., *Seduction of the Innocent* (New York: Rinehart, 1953).

27. White, R., *Ego and Reality in Psychoanalytic Theory* (New York: Int. Univ Press, 1963).

CHAPTER TEN
Mid-Adolescence-Foundations
for Later Psychopathology

Aaron Esman

Adolescence is, by definition, a transitional phase of human psychological development. Whether its duration be brief, as in traditional and "primitive" societies (Muensterberger 1961), or unnaturally extended, as in ours, it looks, Janus-like, back to the childhood past and forward to the adult future. To the extent that it carries the seeds of future pathology, these derive in part from its phase-specific conflicts and developmental issues, and in part from the unresolved problems of early childhood and latency phases and the shadows they cast on the adolescent process.

To understand the foundations and precursors of future psychopathology inherent in the midadolescent period, it is desirable to reconsider the salient issues (or, speaking theologically, "tasks") of this phase as they occur in industrialized societies. The 15-18-year old has, in most cases, experienced the major impact of the physiological changes of puberty. He (or she) has experienced the rebelliousness and turmoil which Offer (1969) acknowledges are characteristic of most early adolescents and which Anna Freud (1958) maintains are a necessary aspect of the adolescent experience. He is well into the throes of object removal and has, in his first postpubertal forays, shifted his major object investments to his peers and to idealized "crush" figures, typically from the world of sport or show business. In his early gropings toward sexual objects he may have enjoyed some experimental homosexual play but is by now reaching out to heterosexual partners, however tentatively. These heterosexual objects are, however, perceived largely on narcissistic lines-"I love what I would like to be," as Blos (1962) formulates it. Life is lived locally and for the moment, although the growth of operational thought (Piaget 1969) is preparing the way for experimentation with abstract concepts and for a wider view of life and its future possibilities.

The passage into mid-adolescence is in many ways analogous to that from Mahler's "hatching" subphase of separation-individuation to the "practicing" period. The 15-18-year-old has acquired an impressive array of new capacities and resources-biological and psychological-which he is now ready to deploy in his interactions with the world around him and in the enhancement of his inner world as well. Erikson (1956) has subsumed much of the work of this subphase under the process of "identity formation." This includes such matters as the establishment of a sexual identity as masculine or feminine (as opposed to gender identity as male or female, which is settled in early childhood) and of a capacity for mutuality in relations with others, particularly with heterosexual partners.

A further component of this process is the development of an orientation to the future, in particular, toward vocational opportunities and choices. This may involve the trying out, either mentally or physically, of alternatives, an aspect of the critical tendency of midadolescents to rest the possibilities that the world offers them. Not the least important among these is the range of possible value orientations; both the aspirations and aims of the ego ideal and the prohibitions of the superego are subject to review and reorganization during adolescence.

All of these phenomena occur in the context of the major task of adolescent development-the process of object removal. Made urgent by the reactivation of oedipal wishes and fears, this process entails the ultimate resolution of dependence-independence conflicts as well as of the incestuous longings and castration anxieties that inhere in the oedipal triangle. In a large sense, it is in the arena of this struggle that many of the aforementioned concerns are settled. By age 18, most of this work will normally have been done; it is left to the stages of late adolescence and (that artifact of our times) "youth" to consolidate the advances that have occurred during the high school years. And it should not be forgotten that for many-perhaps, still, most-young people, high school graduation marks the end of adolescence in most respects and the initiation of adult life.

Unfortunately, as Winnicott (1965) has said, "...some individuals are too ill (with psychoneurosis or depression or schizophrenia) to reach a stage of emotional development that could be called adolescence or they can reach it only in a highly distorted way." For these, the roots of future psychopathology lie in the unresolved conflicts and developmental deviations of earlier periods. For others, the normative developmental events of adolescence proper offer the potentiality for faulty resolution and maladaptive solutions. It is these situations we shall examine here, seeking to delineate some of the intrinsic, the familial, and the social factors that may contribute to such deviant outcome It must be understood, however, that development is a continuous process; the seams in its web are imposed by the observer seeking to order his data into conceptual segments.

Maturational Delays and the Body-Image Problem

By age 15, most adolescents will, as mentioned earlier, have passed through puberty as a physiological process. Especially this is true of girls, some boys on the slow side of the bell-shaped curve may still experience pubertal changes in their 16th year. For them, however, as for that small number whose puberty is delayed beyond the norm, substantial problems arise with both short-term and long-term consequences.

Schoenfeld (1969) has set forth in detail the bodily changes in adolescence and the immediate consequences for body-image formation of deviations from the norm. He stresses the fact that, for adolescents, "to be different is to be inferior." The 15-year-old boy who is forced into invidious dressing-room comparisons of his genital size and pubic hair development with his more biologically favored peers is likely, in order to protect his self-esteem, to withdraw from such situations; he thus risks further stigmatization as a "faggot" or a "bookworm." At least a measure of social awkwardness, at most a pattern of detachment and discomfort in social intercourse may be psychological consequences of such physiological disparity.

The problem of body-image disturbance is even greater among adolescent girls. This can be accounted for by a variety of factors, both sociocultural and intrapsychic. Ours is a culture that imposes on young women, through the mass media, demands for conformity to thoroughly unrealistic standards of bodily form-long-legged, pencil-thin, large-bosomed-that are the despair of most adolescent girls and the delight of the magazines they devour to advise them in their desperate efforts to achieve the unachievable. (The prevailing ethos is manifest in the slogan "There are two things it's impossible to be-too rich or too thin.") At the same time, the normal secondary sexual characteristics are consciously or unconsciously associated with burgeoning sexuality which may, particularly in certain family contexts, be a source of intense shame and/or guilt.

Such conditions may pave the way for one of the most flamboyant disorders of young women-anorexia nervosa. Often setting in during the midadolescent phase, it occurs with equal frequency in late adolescence or young adulthood. Bruch (1973) has defined the multiple determinants of this complex and baffling disorder; prominent among them are disturbances of body image and self-perception (often related to earlier traumata as well as adolescent irregularities). The role of sexual conflicts has been less stressed in Bruch's work than in earlier discussions (Waller, Kauffman, and Deutsch 1940) but should not be overlooked. Unconscious equation of "fat" and "pregnant" and oral impregnation fantasies are common findings in such cases and interdigitate with the separation-individuation and body-image issues emphasized by Bruch and by Sours (1969).

The counter part of such conflictual disturbances in body image is the narcissistic over-investment characteristic of certain hysterical character types. Here, although crucial predispositions may be laid down in earlier phases, adolescence may be the point of crystallization. The adolescent girl requires affirmation of a femininity which is an aspect of her total personality development In particular, she requires acceptance and encouragement from the primary male figures in her life, especially a father who can respond to her growing sexuality with neither defensive withdrawal nor seductive acting out. The integration of sexuality as but one element in a total self-system allows for the enlargement of self-esteem from a variety of intellectual, interpersonal, and conflict-free sources. Where such alternative sources are lacking, the adolescent girl may seek reassurance from excessive (at times monolithic) attention to her appearance and in the development of styles of seductive exhibitionism. Should this be consolidated by parental support or peer approval, the nucleus for later character pathology will be well formed by the end of high school.

Depression and Its Analogs

If the central theme in midadolescence is the pursuit of object removal, it follows that at certain points, a state of relative objectlessness will prevail in the adolescent's mental life. Detaching his emotional engagement from ("decathecting") the mental representations of his parents, he has not yet succeeded in replacing them with stable alternative figures. Much of his activity during these years is devoted to the quest for such attachment objects; for some, this process is fraught with difficulty and frustration. For the adolescent who is shy or temperamentally slow to warm up (Chess, Thomas, and Birch 1967) or for whom early oral disappointments have led to impairments in "basic trust" (Erikson 1950), or whose characterological style is passive, rather than active (Rapaport 1953), the restoration of abandoned object ties may prove an insuperable task. Chronic and lifelong feelings of loneliness and isolation may ensue with a depressive orientation toward life. The fragility of those attachments that are established, and the overinvestment in them as sources of refuge from feelings of loneliness, may lead to major depression and suicidal acts when and if they are disrupted by circumstance or by active disengagement by the partner.

The more-or-less ubiquitous depressive potential in adolescence is normally warded off in a variety of ways. Among these are frenetic hypermotility and social hunger with overtones of hypomanic denial and the use of chemical agents-alcohol and drugs. For most adolescents, these activities are transitory, experimental, and self-limited. For the most vulnerable ones, however, the use of alcohol and drugs may serve as permanent anodynes against the pains of objectlessness. Addiction or drug abuse may, therefore, be among the potential pathologies resident in the miscarried process of object removal (Wieder and Kaplan 1969).

Sexual Identity

Although as noted earlier, gender identity appears to be laid down in the pre-oedipal years, a clear sense of self as masculine or feminine and one's mode of function in one's sexual life are a, product of the adolescent process. Several currents contribute to the ultimate emergence of this configuration. Important among these is the fortification of early identifications by new ones, especially with peer-group members and idealized parent surrogates (not least, those supplied by the mass media). In the resolution of recrudescent oedipal conflicts, such fortifying identifications are crucial, both in promoting the movement toward nonincestuous objects and in buttressing the negative oedipal identification with the same-sex parent.

A crucial aspect of sexual development and of the formation of sexual identity is masturbation. Masturbation is the primary sexual experience of adolescents in our culture, even in this period of "sexual revolution" (Esman 1979). It is vital resource in aiding the adolescent in organizing his sexual fantasies and in permitting experimentation with the pregenital and perverse wishes that can ultimately be integrated into the foreplay of genital heterosexuality. The capacity to masturbate alone and with relative freedom from guilt, is as Borowitz (1973) has pointed out, an essential acquisition in the adolescent's progress towards maturity (cf. the case of Mike).

Potentialities for deviant outcome abound, of course, in so complex a process. As with other aspects discussed here, earlier predispositions play a critical role in determining the outcome of the phase-specific conflicts. Deviant early identifications, particularly those involving intense bisexual ties, will tend to skew the picture and leave the, adolescent open to current influences that may have critical shaping force.

Don F. had emerged from latency with clear male identity but with a complex pattern of identifications with a powerful, overbearing, "phallic" mother and remote critical father who offered him little protection or support. His longing for an internalized sense of masculine power could be gratified only by oral incorporation. Seduced in early adolescence by an older male friend of the family into performing fellatio, he came to use this means to seduce his peers from whom he sought not sexual gratification per se, but friendship and acceptance. This pattern became consolidated during his high school years so that by 17 he was a confirmed, though but highly conflicted homosexual. Fantasies of biting off the penis represented not only his wish to incorporate the phallus and to gain its power, but a persistent identification with the devouring, castrating mother.

Leslie T. was a depressed, somewhat bewildered 21.year-old girl, fresh out of a prestigious women's college and uncertain about her direction in life. Her sadness was a reaction to the departure for Europe of a young woman who had been her homosexual lover through 3 college years. Leslie's family situation was bizarre. Her father lived and worked in a Midwestern city. Her mother had taken Leslie and her 2-year older brother to live in Florida when Leslie was 12, and the father came for occasional visits and vacations. Mrs. T. was a vain, narcissistic woman who was completely idle and emotionally detached from her children. Leslie grew up an unhappy, object-hungry girl who at 15 formed a homosexual liaison with a classmate, which coexisted with heterosexual friendships and dates. In this relationship, and in the subsequent one in college, her aim was clearly to be cared for and mothered by a warm, dominant lover.

On the other hand, Blos (1957) has described the type of adolescent girl who takes flight into precocious and promiscuous heterosexuality from the unconscious pull toward an erotized tie to the pre-oedipal mother. In her eagerness to disavow such longings, tinged as they are with homosexual and infantile dependent meanings, such a girl becomes, Blos says, a "Diana," intent on pursuing her masculine prey with pseudosexual seductions. Others, with conflicts and motives similar to Leslie's, will turn their erotic attention to males as well, seeking from them maternal care rather than mature heterosexual mutuality. In adult life such women are likely to experience repeated failures in their love lives or to immerse themselves in masochistic dependence on men to whom they remain attached, despite repeated disappointments and/or sadistic manipulation, out of their terror of abandonment and loneliness. Beating fantasies may appear in such women; behind the sadistic male figure in such fantasies is the rejecting angry mother of pre-oedipal times.

Future Orientation and Work Goals

Prior to mid-adolescence, children are essentially present oriented, at first because of the immaturity of their cognitive organization and their dependence on adults and, in early adolescence, because of the intensity of their narcissism and their primary preoccupation with puberty and its consequences. In the high school years this begins to change. The cognitive development described by Piaget (op. cit.) permits a broader awareness of the nature of the world and the possibilities it affords, and the realities of adult life. The emergence from pubertal narcissism in the direction of more substantial object attachments serves further to foster anticipation of adult sexual role requirements. And the growing consolidation of identifications, positive or negative, engenders vocational interests attuned to them as well as to emerging intrinsic interests and talents in the adolescent, at least the range of vocational possibilities is broad and allows for the accommodation of individual tastes, interests, and special capacities. Premature closure, unreflective decisions based on defensive identifications or avoidance intended to obviate anxiety, or due to ideological commitments attendant on ego-ideal reshaping (Erikson's 'absolutism'), or submissive conformity to parental demands and pressures-all may lead to lifelong dissatisfaction or to repeated changes of vocational role in later life.

Alternatively, the adolescent who is too closely tied to his primary objects, who fears detaching himself and establishing his own identity, or who, due to parental overindulgence, is unwilling to relinquish the infantile dependent position may avoid engaging in the business of experimentation with and exploration of work possibilities. Locked into a passive posture, he may either defer such choices endlessly and assume the position of "prolonged adolescence" described by Bernfeld (1938) or he may settle submissively into a predetermined situation unrelated to his own gifts.

It must be acknowledged that forces exist in the contemporary world that promote such prolongation of adolescence. What Erikson has called the "psychosocial moratorium"-that period during which society allows for experimentation and deferral of commitment-has been funkier and funkier extended in recent decades, with the prolongation of the period of education demanded of young people and with the need to keep at least the more affluent among them out of the labor force as long as feasible. For some, the absence of external pressure to end this moratorium resonates with inner passivity and dependency wishes to produce a type of prolonged adolescence characterized by the "hippies" of the 1960s, the peripatetic remittance man, and the interminable graduate student. If to this is added the failure to resolve the renascent oedipal conflicts, potency difficulties and/or flight from commitment to sexual objects will complete the syndrome.

Ego Synthesis and the Management of Regression

The traditional picture of normal adolescent development would have it that puberty initiates a prolonged period of instability and turmoil, marked by multiple and shifting regressions and progressions in drive and ego organization until, somewhere in late adolescence, a process of synthesis and coalescence takes place that engenders the stable ego and character organization of adult life. Only in recent years have workers such as Masterson (1968) and Offer (op. cit.) challenged this view, setting forth evidence suggesting that the turmoil ridden adolescent is a disturbed adolescent and that most young people negotiate the high school years without major disruption of personality integrity.

That this is the case does not, of course, minimize the stresses of the mid-adolescent period, it suggests, rather, that most young people bring to them a system of defenses and coping capacities that enable them successfully to weather these stresses. It is well known, however, that a significant number cannot do so. For those that bring to this phase a fragile ego, the burdens of individuation on the one hand (Masterson 1973) and the establishment of intimate object ties on the other (Erikson 1950) may prove insuperable.

The vulnerable adolescent faced with such threats may break down completely, evidencing an acute psychotic disorder which may, or in rare cases may not, be the prelude to long-term schizophrenic illness. In order to maintain a semblance of integrity, however, he will more frequently protect his tenuous psychic structure by withdrawing into a schizoid isolation, communing in dereistic fantasies with the introjected-and at times, projected-figures of his infantile objects.

Jim R., 16 years old, was referred to me after he had just dropped out of college during the Christmas vacation of his freshman year. For the month before the break he had been avoiding classes, sleeping during the day and awake at night. preoccupied with ideas about precognition and psychokinesis.

Mathematically gifted, he was determined that he could find a way to forecast the vagaries of the stock market and predict the winners of horse races- indeed, to determine these events by the power of his own thoughts. By the time he came to see me he had some awareness of the irrationality of these ideas, but he was still occupied with them and oscillated between belief and skepticism.

Jim was the only child of relatively elderly parents, who doted on him and were gratified by his intellectual precocity. He had been overprotected in early childhood, and his earliest memory was of his acute anxiety and tearfulness when he was put on a bus to go to day camp at age 5 or 6. Academically, school had posed no problems for him and he coasted through quickly with little or no effort; his grades declined in his last year in high school but not enough to preclude his admission to a high-prestige college. His matriculation there marked the first time he had ever been away from home for any extended period. He had always "hung out" with peer groups in his neighborhood, but had no intimate friends. Though fascinated by girls and involved in ruminations about social and sexual triumphs, he had never really dated a girl before he left for college.

Thus Jim was confronted by a succession of stressful circumstances on entering college. Not only did he have to cope with separation from his overinvolved parents, but he was thrust into dormitory life, which imposed on him demands for closeness with peers and simultaneously threatened his shaky sexual identity. Further, his somewhat grandiose narcissism felt the shock of the more stringent academic pressures and his rapid realization that he was no longer the boy wonder he had been in high school.

The result was a breakdown and regression in multiple areas of ego function; his emergency defense was largely that of intellectualization and a reinforcement of other obsessive compulsive defenses- a desperate effort to control his world by means of thought. Removal from the traumatic situation and return home provided rapid relief, but it was only after several months of intensive therapy that his thinking became more reality-bound and that he was able to take a job preparatory to returning to a local university the next year. He lost one job because of persistent lateness and lack of commitment, and his first return to college was similarly unsuccessful. The second time he set up an easy schedule and seemed able to function at adequate but marginal level. He continued in therapy until he was almost 19. Although there was no indication of further psychotic thinking or behavior, his character became consolidated into a rather shallow, narcissistic one with a focus on the quick solution and the "easy buck."

Ego Ideal and Superego Development

As Blos (1974) and Esman (1972) have recently pointed out, adolescence affords an opportunity for the reshaping of the ego ideal and a readjustment of the superego. More closely attuned to current reality, closer to consciousness, and normally less peremptory in nature, the former is likely to undergo more extensive reorganization on the basis of new identifications. Much of the psychological activity of adolescence is related to the revamping of the value system; the constant experimentation of adolescents with values alternative to or in conflict with those of their parents or of the dominant cultural ethos reflects not merely "rebellion" but a genuine effort to find and formulate a self-syntonic system of values. The oft-described decline in the credibility of traditional sources of values (cf. e.g., Esman 1977) makes this process all the more urgent and all the more difficult.

The superego (in the restricted sense as the store of prohibitive and self-critical values) also undergoes some modification. Certainly, it loses its categorical, all-or-none quality, as the evolving cognitive system allows for more shadings and concessions to reality (Nass 1966). The earlier absolute prohibitions against sexual activity, for instance, are adjusted to the adolescent's new needs and capacities. Normally the incest taboo is not only maintained but fortified, although incestuous fantasies are not unusual, even in consciousness.

It is precisely with regard to this adaptation to current and future reality that the potential for later pathology resides. Although the ultimate consolidation of the ego ideal and superego is the work of late adolescence, the way is paved during the midadolescent period. Preservation of archaic value-centered introjects (Sandler 1960) threatens the maintenance of self-esteem under conditions of stress, with both shame and guilt as irrational and potentially self-damaging consequences. Thus the failure to adjust narcissistically tinged introjections of overevaluated parent figures may induce totally unrealizable grandiose or omnipotent goals. The college student who fails to achieve in conformity with such goals (or even worse, who fails in the course of his desperate efforts to do so) may react with acute depression, feelings of hopelessness, and even suicide. Similarly, adolescents who fail to resolve sexual prohibitions, including those against masturbation, may emerge with lifelong sexual conflicts which may lead to acting out of perverse or deviant fantasies in ostensibly nonsexual ways.

Mike, a 19-year-old college junior came to treatment because of chronic feelings of self-doubt and inferiority and intense social and sexual anxieties. Born to a rich family, reared in an exclusive suburb, educated in expensive private schools, he appeared slovenly and unkempt, with holes in his trousers, long shaggy hair, and a droopy blond moustache. He was a former drug user, having had 3 or 4 years. Regular experience with marijuana and LSD and the values attending them before abruptly abandoning them completely after a "bad trip' during which he almost jumped out of a window.

Mike's sexual inhibitions were profound. He was extremely shy with women, constantly concerned about sexual performance, and generally experienced premature ejaculation in coitus. He elaborated complex, compensatory fantasies of sexual triumph associated with situations in which, as a radical political leader, he would be jailed or hospitalized, achieving through his martyrdom reconciliation with his conservative parents and amatory successes with beautiful young women devoted to his political cause. For a long period during his analysis, Mike insisted that he had never masturbated before he was 17. Gradually, however, it became clear that he was referring to manual masturbation. In fact, from age 14 he had masturbated by rubbing his genitals against his bed sheets while in a prone position. This, however, he did not consider masturbation, i.e., he was able to carry on this activity while at the same time denying what he was doing because of his profound feelings of guilt and shame, related in part to conscious incestuous fantasies about his sister. The inhibitions implicit in this pattern were clearly expressed in his sexual symptoms. His fantasies, however, with their passive, masochistic character, similarly served as continuing expressions of the masturbatory fantasies of his early arid mid-adolescent years.

In contrast, Johnson (1949) described situations in which parental sanction or complicity generated superego defects or "lacunae" that may portend long lasting character pathology. "The child's superego lacunae correspond to similar defects of the parents' superegos which in turn were derived from the conscious or unconscious permissiveness of their own parents." Such persons will demonstrate focal deviation from culturally shared norms of behavior *without* intrapsychic conflict.

It is apparent then, that the mid-adolescent period is of crucial significance in the evolution of adult personality. As Giovacchini (1973) puts it, "...the adult personality is psychopathologically construed insofar as it is the outcome of reactions against what has been *experienced* as a traumatic adolescence." (italics mine) The person's *experience* of adolescence will reflect not only the observable realities of his life situation, but also the personality structure and characteristics he brings to them. It is, of course, commonplace for patients- and nonpatients-to ascribe the "traumatic" or stressful quality of their adolescence, whether current or remembered, to external circumstances-not least, parents, teachers, or other adults. It is well to recall that the picture one receives is filtered through the veil of retrospective distortion and influenced by the persistence of primitive object representations and of introjective- projective defenses that make the reconstruction of adolescent experience particularly difficult in adult analysis. "We fail," says Anna Freud (1958), "to recover...the atmosphere in which the adolescent lives..." What remains for most adults is a profound sense that it was a period they would not want to live through again. "Experience tells us," says Blos (1977), "that unresolved psychological issues are always bound to remain; it is, however, their stable integration into the adult personality that gives these persistent issues a pattern and rather irreversible structure." For some, unfortunately, this pattern, this irreversibility, takes on pathological form.

References

Bernfeld, S. Types of adolescents. *Psychoanalytic Quarterly,* 7:243-253, 1938.

Blos, P. Precedipal factors in the etiology of female delinquency. *The Psychoanalytic Study of the Child,* 12:229- 249, 1957.

On Adolescence: A Psychoanalytic Interpretation. New York:Free Press of Glencoe, 1962.

269 pp.

The genealogy of the ego ideal. *The Psychoanalytic Study of the Child,* 24:43-88, 1974.

When and how does adolescence end? In: Feinstein, S.C., and Giovacchini, P., eds. *Adolescent Psychiatry.* Vol. 5. New York: Aronson, 1977. pp. 5-17.

Borowitz, G. The capacity to masturbate alone. In: Feinstein, S.C., and Giovacchini, P., eds. *Adolescent Psychiatry.* Vol.2. New York: Basic Books, 1973.

Bruch, H. *Eating Disorders.* New York: Basic Books, 1973.

Chess, S.; Thomas, A; and Birch, H. Behavior problems revisited: Findings of an anterospenive study. *Journal of the American Academy of Child Psychiatry,* 6:321-331, 1967.

Erikson, E.H. Growth and crises of the healthy personality. In: Senn, M.J.E.ed. *Symposium on the Healthy Personality, Supp. II. Transactions of the 4th Annual Conference on Problems of Infancy and Childhood.* New York: Josiah ,Macy Foundation, 1950. pp. 91-146.

The problem of ego identity. *Journal of the American Psychoanalytic Association,* 4:56-121, 1956.

Esman, A H. Adolescence and the consolidation of values. In: Post, S.C., ed. *Moral Values and the Superego Concept in Psychoanalysis.* New York

International Universities Press, 1972.
Changing values: Their implications for adolescent development and psychoanalytic ideas. In: Feinstein, S.C., and Giovacchini, P., eds. *Adolescent Psychiatry* Vol. 5. New York Aronson, 1977, pp. 18-34.
Adolescence and the "New Sexuality."' In: Karasu, T., and Socarides, C.R., eds. *On Sexuality: Psychoanalytic Observations.*New York: International Universities Press, 1979. pp. 19-28.
Freud, A. Adolescence. *The Psychoanalytic Study of the Child*, 13:255-278, 1958.
Giovacchini, P. The adolescent process and character formation: Clinical aspects. In: Feinstein., S.C., and Giovacchini, P., eds. *Adolescent Psychiatry.* Vol. 2. New York Basic Books, 1973. pp. 269-285.
Johnson, A. Sanctions for superego lacunae of adolescents. In: Eissler, K.R., ed. *Searchlights on Delinquency.* New York: International Universities Press, 1949. pp. 225-245.
Masterson,J. The psychiatric significance of adolescent turmoil. *American Journal of Psychiatry*, 124(11):1549- 1554, 1968.
The borderline adolescent. In: Feinstein, S.C., and Giovacchini, P., eds. *Adolescent Psychiatry.* Vol. 2. New York Basic Books, 1973.
Muensterberger, W. The adolescent in society. In: Lorand, S., and Schnees, H., eds. *Adolescence.* New York: Paul B. Hoeber, 1961.
Nass, M. The superego and moral development in the theories of Freud and Piaget. *The Psychoanalytic Study of the Child*, 21:51-68, 1966.
Offer, D. *The Psychological World of the Teenager.* New York Basic Books, 1969.
Piaget, J. The intellectual development of the adolescent. In: Caplan, G., and Lebovici, S., eds. *Adolescence, Psychosocial Perspectives* New York: Basic Books, 1969. pp. 22-26.
Rapaport, D. Some metapsychological considerations concerning activity and passivity (1953). In: Gill, M.M.. ed. *Collected Papers of David Rapaport.* New York Basic Books, 1967.
Sandler.J. On the concept of superego. *The Psychoanalytic Study of the Child*, 15:128- 162, 1960.
Schoenfeld. W. The body and the body image. In: Caplan, G., and Lebovici, S., eds. *Adolescence, Psychosocial Perspectives.* New   York: Basic Books, 1969.
Sours, J. Anorexia nervosa: Nosology, diagnosis, development process and power-control mechanisms. In: Caplan. G.. and Lebovici, S.. eds. *Adolescence, Psychosocial Perspectives.* New York: Basic Books, 1969.

Waller, J.V.; Kaufman. M.R.: and Deutsch. F. Anorexia nervosa: A psychosomatic entity. *Psychosomatic Medicine*, 2:3- 16, 1940.
Wieder, H., and Kaplan. E. Drug use in adolescents: Psvchodynamic meaning and pharmacogenic effect. *The Psychoanalytic Study of the Child*, 14:399-451, 1969.
Winnicott, D. Adolescence: Struggling through the doldrums. In: *The Family and Individual Development*. New York: Basic Books. 1965.

CHAPTER ELEVEN
LATE ADOLESCENCE: DEVELOPMENTAL AND CLINICAL CONSIDERATIONS

Samuel Ritvo

Puberty and adolescence usher in a period of rapid physiological, morphological, and psychological change normally lasting 6 to 8 years. The psychoanalytic elucidation of this kaleidoscopic period has gained enormously from the approach of dividing adolescence into stages and defining each phase by its phenomenological characteristics and the corresponding metapsychological conceptualizations. In this way we have progressed in our knowledge of the instinctual upheaval, the shifts in object relations, alternations between regression and progression, and the restructuring of the psychic apparatus, all of which underlie the otherwise baffling phenomenology of adolescence.

Late adolescence is important to distinguish as a stage because it defines that period at the end of adolescence when the last major spontaneous integration and structuring of the personality takes place as the adolescent enters upon the psychological and reality tasks of adult life. Blos (1962) stresses that unlike puberty and early adolescence when rapid morphological and physiological changes occur, the closing phase of adolescence can be defined only by its psychological features. It is a period of development in which no new intrinsic maturational or biological energies enter the picture. But the psychological features of late adolescence do reflect the fact that this is the age when the biologically mature individual must take steps defining who he is in relation to his society. The duration and style of adolescence are influenced more by cultural and social factors than any other developmental period. The start is determined biologically by puberty; but it may be prolonged by internal psychic conditions in the individual and by the conditions of society. This period spans what Erikson (1956) has described as the psychosocial moratorium. In our post-industrial technological society this period is more prolonged for more individuals who comprise a greater segment of society

This paper was presented as the Brill Memorial Lecture at the New York Academy of Medicine, November 24, 1970. From the Child Study Center, Yale University.

than in previous historical periods. The transition to work and love in the realistic world is a longer process.   As psychoanalysts we probably have our largest and most intensive experience with that segment of the youth population which is most affected by the conditions which prolong adolescence -the subsidized, dependent student group. With the vastly increased size of this group it seems likely that more persons are drawn into this group who are not suited to a life in which inner organization and motivation are at a premium and in which immediate reality demands closer to self-preservation do not support the ego in its autonomy from the instinctual drives.

What are the main developmental issues of late adolescence? Blos (1962) stresses that late adolescence is primarily a phase of consolidation in which there is an "elaboration of: 1) a highly idiosyncratic and stable arrangement of ego functions and interests; 2) an extension of the conflict-free sphere of the ego (secondary autonomy); 3) an irreversible sexual position (identity constancy); 4) a relatively constant cathexis of object- and self-representations; and 5) the stabilization of mental apparatuses which automatically safeguard the integrity of the psychic organism" (p. 129). In a later paper (1967), Blos examines further the relationship between the consolidation of psychic structure and character formation as a normative integrative process aimed at the elimination of conflict and anxiety arousal. He assigns to this process primarily a regulatory function in the maintenance of homeostasis in patterned self-esteem regulation, in the stabilization of ego identity (Erikson, 1956), in the automatization of threshold and barrier levels to internal and external stimuli, and in the containment of affective fluctuations, including depression, within a tolerable range.

Jacobson (1964) lays great stress on the changes in the ego and superego identifications of the adolescent. In late adolescence, an unmistakable shift of power to the ego occurs which gives it increasing influence on id and superego. The ego acquires the role of an active mediator. The adolescent's worldly strivings and his identifications with the realistic images of his parents are used as aids for the readjustments of the superego and its moral codes. The superego enters into a new equilibrium with the id and ego in which the id is restricted and more mature ego goals and standards of achievement are adopted. The formation and structuralization of the ego ideal are crucial developmental steps in adolescence.

The modifications in the psychic systems in late adolescence stem from a confluence of social and reality pressures on the one hand and internal strivings on the other. The crises of late adolescence arise because of the failure to achieve the earlier developmental tasks, especially the failure to resolve the effects of childhood neuroses and other developmental disturbances which have distorted the ego and hampered the development of object relations. The increasing demands on the ego toward the end of adolescence to take the ascendancy in the last spontaneous integration and consolidation of the personality may bring long-standing, latent vulnerabilities of the ego into open clinical manifestation. The clinical crises of this period span the full range of character disorders, psychoneuroses, and borderline conditions. It is also the age of greatest liability to the severest failures of the ego, the psychoses. The crises of personality integration present themselves in terms of the life issues of the period: the difficulties in approaching the new heterosexual object; the concerns about homosexuality; the reactions to the inexorable processes of self-definition as these go forward in choices and decisions determined by the past as well as the present and the visions of the future.

The individual in crisis responds intrapsychically to the conflict over these issues along the pathways prepared by his earlier development in terms of anxiety, regression, defense, and symptom formation. The dynamics of these conflicts do not change basically from generation to generation and follow the basic psychological laws that govern intrapsychic phenomena. Yet the manifest expression of these conflicts does change because a person can use only the vehicles at hand in the contemporary historical period of his society and culture or those which he invents using the modalities at hand in his environment. When the vehicles at hand include drugs, new methods of contraception, worldwide instant communications, jet-age mobility, the threat of nuclear explosions, and a technological society in which adolescence is prolonged, the conditions exist for such kaleidoscopic shifts in available life styles and such distorted or apparently novel behavioral expressions of basic psychological conflicts that their recognition as variations of basic themes may be hampered for a time. There still remains the possibility that such extensive external changes and the changing moral attitudes which are internalized bring about more than "apparent" change. Furthermore, in treating individuals the analyst always deals with the variations rather than the basic theme.

Of the many factors entering into the crises of late adolescence I would like to examine in more detail two which play an important part in this period-object relations and ego-ideal formation-and therefore also have an impact on the technique of psychoanalysis during this period. My discussion is limited to the male because my analytic experience in recent years has been preponderantly with males. I hope that the advent of coeducation at Yale will help to correct this and teach us more about the salient differences between male and female adolescent development.

Object Relations

In early adolescence the reawakened pregenital urges and the newly acquired genital urges are in danger of making contact with the libidinal cathexes of the original objects from the oedipal and preoedipal past (Anna Freud, 1958). This lends a new and threatening reality to hitherto repressed fantasies. The anxiety which arises becomes a motive force in the efforts to loosen or break the ties to the infantile objects. The breaking of the object ties and the return of the libido to the self and the ego result in the increased narcissism of the adolescent. The heightened narcissistic libido manifests itself in the bodily preoccupations, the hypochondriacal tendencies, and the prominence of somatizations in the psychoneurotic symptoms of adolescence. The quickly established and often equally quickly broken attachments to peers and adults are formed on the basis of idealizations which are externalizations and projections of the adolescent's own narcissism. These relationships are the basis for new identifications and are initial steps in the reversal of libidinal cathexis from the self to the object but do not yet constitute lasting new object ties.

The late adolescent must leave his narcissistic retreat and turn more to the external world for gratification and self-realization, a process that has major consequences for his relationship to the external world. Paradoxically, with the establishment of genital primacy, the individual becomes directly dependent on the body of the object in a way that has not existed since infancy. This can be seen in the strong bodily and emotional ties that the individual has to the person with whom he experiences the genital sexual gratification. The greater dependence for gratification upon the external object brings about a shift in the relations or balance between the reality principle and the pleasure principle. Reality now assumes a relatively greater role in the attainment of pleasure than it previously had. The role of fantasy is relatively lessened and assumes more preparatory and anticipatory functions.

With the progress of adolescence the individual shifts from gratification or discharge largely in connection with fantasy about the object to gratification more directly in activity with the object.

The adolescent is impelled in this shift by his own more intense erotic arousal and object hunger which press him to function according to the reality principle in the service of the pleasure principle. Attempts at gratification through fantasy prove disappointing to the adolescent just as attempts toward hallucinatory gratification proved disappointing in the past. Unlike the infant who does not know at first that the external object is necessary and responds with crying and helplessness, the adolescent knows that the external object is necessary and seeks the object. In both there is no fully adequate substitute for the external object.

The younger child is predominantly in a passive position in relation to the object, whereas the adolescent is much more in an active role. The necessary and phase-specific turn to activity with the external object means that the sexual excitement which was previously discharged in fantasy and the autoplastic activity of masturbation now has to seek gratification in the context of the alloplastic relationship to the external object. For the adolescent this constitutes a new and strange reality element to be mastered. One consequence of the turn toward greater activity is the increased possibility of anxiety and conflict over the discharge of aggression upon the object, requiring the institution of vigorous defenses or avoidance or flight from the object.

Another consequence of the turn toward the external object in the move toward the genital sexual relationship is that the conditions of pleasure gain for the individual become more manifest and more specific. As the conditions of pleasure gain dictate the situations and practices which enhance or inhibit sexual excitement and responsiveness, the adolescent becomes aware of the limitations and distortions of his sexual life over which he has little or no control. The conditions of pleasure gain have multiple internal sources. They arise from the conditions of infantile sexual life (Freud, 1914): from the quantitative aspect of the component instincts, indicating the fixation points of earlier libidinal and aggressive development; from object relations, dictating the characteristics of the partner; or from the superego, necessitating guilt and self-punitive or self-damaging behavior.

When the adolescent turns to the external object, the fantasies which were a source of pleasure in connection with masturbation may become a source of acute conflict when the gratification has to be sought directly with the object and not exclusively in fantasy. Early in adolescence when the new genital urges and the reawakened pregenital strivings connect with the oedipal and preoedipal objects, the fantasies were a source of anxiety because they threatened to become too realistic. In later adolescence when the realistic relationship with the new object is taken up, the individual has to cope with the revival of the libidinal cathexes of the old objects as they appear now in the context of the realistic relationship. The necessity to *act upon* the old oedipal and preoedipal fantasies becomes a source of increased anxiety. The nuclear infantile conflicts come up for final resolution, so to speak, with the difference that there is a greater element of reality to conflicts which earlier had existed largely in fantasy.

Eissler (1958) has examined the function of orgasm in adolescence in the fusion of the unconscious representation of reality with the specific external circumstances. He emphasizes the first orgasm in puberty and the establishment of orgasm in a permanent place in the life of the adolescent as crucial experiences in the long developmental process by which the reality principle is installed and maintained in psychic life.

To the ego already distorted, restricted or split by infantile and childhood conflict and experience; to the superego which has not been modified by influence from a normally functioning ego, the situation becomes acute and may assume critical proportions. The time to choose a life work and make a commitment cannot be staved off further, the young man's measure will finally be taken for all the world to know. The oedipal conflict comes to life in earnest for the time has actually come to take the man's place. The issue may become particularly transparent in those young men who enter their father's profession or vocation, and a frequent point of breakdown is on taking this step in school. The unconscious death wishes against the oedipal rival regain a poignancy absent since the height of the oedipal period. The shift of influence to the ego also means that the ego reacts more intensely to these dystonic elements in the form of anxiety, symptom formation, and concern for the future of the work life and love relationships. This is often the point at which the adolescent comes for treatment.

The path from the first new approaches to the object in adolescence to the adult love relationship involving lasting intimacy and care is a developmental process extending over a period of years. Although the pleasure principle impels the adolescent to turn actively to the new object for gratification, the object choice and the object relationship have at first *both* narcissistic and anaclitic elements. In his approach to the new object the adolescent starts from the position of ego regression described by Geleerd (1961) in which he gives signs of regression to the undifferentiated phase of object relations with wishes and fantasies of merging with the object and blurring of the ego boundaries.

Geleerd viewed this regression as necessary for later healthy ego integration in the adolescent. I am interested here in the steps by which the adolescent emerges from this regressed position. Even in the heterosexual object the male adolescent can love what he once was or would like to be. The object is often seen as embodying ideals he has for himself in qualities of mind and body and the incandescent passion may flicker and go out when she does not live up to an ideal he has for himself. She may be regarded as a possession or attribute of the self which can be a source of pride and satisfaction if she is seen as perfect or a source of shame and self-criticism if she is viewed as flawed or defective. The initial steps toward the new object contain elements of the adolescent's own narcissism which can be discerned in the attitudes and behavior toward the new object.

Clinical psychoanalytic observation suggests that for the adolescent the new object serves functions that in some ways resemble those the object had in infancy and early childhood (Kris, 1955). At that time the central love object acts as a stabilizer of physiological and affective processes. Where the central love object is absent as in institutionalized children, Kris hypothesized that the neutralization of instinctual energy does not take place to the usual degree and the ego is not invested with the energies which lead to the normally expected developmental steps such as the organization of action and problem solving even if the noninstinctual energies connected with the maturational processes are available. This old pathway is used again by the adolescent who has retreated to a narcissistic position in the course of loosening the ties to the infantile objects and who is absorbed in himself, his body, his feelings, his thought processes. In this condition he is likely to have somatic and hypochondriacal symptoms, to be preoccupied with existential ruminations about the absurdity of life, to be without a sense of purpose, and to shift rapidly from exalted feelings to feeling worthless. He may be unable to organize himself for action or work if there is no immediate or urgent reality demand, and even this may fail to activate him.

This state may change with dramatic swiftness with the cathexis of the external object. Not only do the manifestations of the narcissistic investment of the self abate with the cathexis of the object, but the capacity to organize for action and work and the sense of purpose and being in touch with the real world are strengthened. The sequence from narcissistic investment to cathexis of the object and then to improved functioning in activities requiring increased supplies of neutralized instinctual energies can be observed repeatedly in the same individual. At these times the object serves again as the mother once served-as an organizer with whom the child identifies, thus making neutralized energies available for development in the direction of sublimation and work.

Although the adolescent turns actively to the object for gratification, he does so with a resurgence of old passive, anaclitic aims toward the object. They take the form of a revival of the old dependent, clinging, possessive demands toward the object with abrupt outbursts of the negative, hostile side of the ambivalence at the slightest rebuff or frustration, which is experienced as a painful, narcissistic wound. During the period of emergence from the narcissistic retreat of earlier adolescence, the relationship to the object shows some of the features of the infantile   relationship to the need-satisfying object.

A central narcissistic concern related to the castration anxiety of the phallic-oedipal phase is the concern over genital potency (Deutsch, 1967). Frequently, it is only after this concern subsides with the establishment of potency that the passive, infantile strivings toward the object come into the foreground. The passive strivings and the need for the object as organizer were expressed succinctly by a sophomore at a time when he was experiencing an insatiable sexual curiosity and desire for everyone he encountered, man or woman. He said, "Wanting girls so much is a weakness because of why I want them. I need a girl for physical stability. I need the warmth, the flesh. I want to be taken in the warm insides of the girl. But I know that aggressive courting is necessary for that and I don't feel up to it at the moment. Smoking marijuana is a good substitute for a girl. It gives me the same feeling of calm fulfillment."

In another hour during the same period of the analysis when he felt that his activities had no significance and that life had no meaning for him he spoke again of his longing for a girl. "A girl's is my link with the world. I can't touch anything until I touch a girl. The world becomes real that way. If I can control the girl's body, it makes my body whole. It is a way to get from my own body to the world. My own body becomes a tool rather than a reflection."

The first approaches to the new object start from a strongly narcissistic position and the active turning to the object is accompanied by an intensification of passive aims. The intensified passive wishes to merge and be taken close revive former anxieties connected with fantasies and fears of engulfment. Through the projection of the aggressive components onto the object and reversal of the passive and dependent strivings the male adolescent views the woman again as a phallic woman who threatens him in a variety of ways still related to the strongly narcissistic investment of his body and his self-image. He is tortured by concerns that she will not find him adequate, that she will deplete him physically, that she will offer temptations which will undermine his resolve to commit himself to a goal. These concerns also contain the hostile and punitive reactions of the superego against the oedipal content of the masturbation fantasies of the antecedent adolescent period. Under these influences the attitude toward the new object oscillates between a feeling of urgent need for a close, exclusive possessive relationship with the heterosexual object and an anxious apprehension that the girl clings to him, makes demands on him, and threatens his freedom and integrity.

The willingness of the girl to enter into such a relationship is for the male adolescent a gratifying and reassuring, though often transitory confirmation of his consolidating realistic sense of his own worth as he moves developmentally from the self image which has been distorted by the narcissistic retreat and the exaggerated intellectual and ascetic defenses of the earlier period of adolescence. The object plays a crucial role as an external referent for the internal reorganization which takes place.

The eventual steps toward lasting intimacy and care are dependent on the ability to progress from the predominantly narcissistic relationship to the object and to tolerate the anaclitic dependence on the object which otherwise has to be avoided by many adolescents because of the painful affects and aggression connected with it from childhood frustrations and disappointments. Normally, both the narcissistic satisfactions and the object libidinal gratifications which can be gained from the new object raise the self-regard of the ego and contribute both to the consolidation of the ego in late adolescence and to a change in the ego ideal in the direction of deriving gratification from being able to realize some parts of the ideal and of being the one to provide for the loved person in a variety of ways. This contributes an element of pleasure gain to the work functions. Genetically the change draws upon oedipal and preoedipal ideals but is also realistically rooted in the new developmental capacity to provide genital sexual pleasure, itself an important source of narcissistic gratification.

The strong impression gained from clinical psychoanalytic observation that passive aims are prominent in the initial approaches to the new object may be colored by a selection factor, since it is quite likely that the more passive adolescents gravitate toward analysis. Nevertheless, this may be an instance again in which the study of pathology or one sector of normal variation may contribute to the understanding of development. When the adolescent takes the first steps in turning actively toward the new object in the developmental move toward the assumption of the adult sexual role and the mature love relationship, he does so only partly in identification with the ideal of the phallic-oedipal period. In large measure he turns to the new object with passive needs as he did to the earlier external object so that the object again functions as an organizer and stabilizer crucial to the consolidation of late adolescence. The interplay between drive and object is essential to the emergence from the narcissistic retreat.

Although the relationship to the new object may have a large narcissistic element in the beginning arid this may be a prerequisite for daring to take the step so risky to his self-esteem, other developmental issues in the resolution of which the object has a role are carried along in this step. The object is also an immediate portion of reality to which the adolescent turns for the nutriment he needs in the looming struggle over what will be his place in life. The object's interest and love are the needed replacements for the blows to his narcissism which the adolescent anticipates and sustains as he makes his choices. His decisions eventually transform the omnipotentiality of the youth (Pumpian-Mindlin, 1965) into the specific, individual, delimited identity of the adult. In this the object functions for the individual in a manner synergistic with and complementary to the ego ideal. As one 19-year-old expressed it, "Sometimes I wonder how good I am compared to the others around me. Most of the time I know I'm pretty good, but I would like to have someone who would be interested enough in me or care enough about me to share what I think and what I feel."

It is well known that identification with the parents in their adult role plays a large part in the shift of power to the ego in late adolescence. But it is important to realize fully the role of the new object in this process of consolidation of the ego because the object offers the possibility both of gratifying the instinctual drives and, via identification with the object as a repetition of the early central love object, making available to the ego increased resources of neutralized instinctual energies for its adaptive functioning.

The actual experience with the object in infancy and early childhood has a profound effect on the outcome of adolescence. The object stands in a pivotal position between the instinctual drives and reality in the reorganization of the drives under the hegemony of the ego in late adolescence. The outcome of this developmental process in adolescence is therefore critically affected by the history, the characteristics, and the experiences of the earlier object relations. This is the time when the effects of deprivation, loss, separation, deficiencies, and peculiarities of mothering which resulted in the developmental disturbances of infancy and early childhood become operative again. Sleep and eating disturbances, somatic complaints and bodily concerns become frequent and are prominent in the symptom formation of this period. The earlier disturbances in object relations may have impaired the development from the need satisfying object to object constancy with resulting deviations and distortions in the ego. These may have a particularly strong impact on children with constitutional vulnerabilities. In the face of the new demands of genital sexuality, of the need to make realistic commitments in the irreversible process of self-definition which threatens the narcissistic self image, the adolescent makes use of old object representations and looks for new objects in the external world who can be merged and blended with the old object representations in the search for the necessary accommodation of both instinctual drives and external reality. The adolescent with early impairment of ego and object relations has severe difficulty making his way back from the ego regression of earlier adolescence.

The recognition of the widening chasm between the defensively aggrandized self image and the desperately struggling self produces intense anxiety and heightened feelings of guilt and shame. The excessive ambivalence and hostility which accompanied the early unsatisfactory object relations now interfere with the capacity to identify with the parental objects in their adult roles and with the new objects on the model of the earlier central love object as stabilizer and organizer. This is after all the age of greatest incidence of schizophrenic psychosis in which there is a break with reality. It is also the time of greatest need for the therapies which provide direct support for the ego through supplying an object, often through specialized communities in institutions.

The Ego Ideal

The consolidation and integration of the ego toward the end of adolescence also occur in consonance with changes in the ego ideal. Because the ego ideal is the substitute for the lost narcissism of the individual's childhood it remains throughout life an agency of the mind which is most closely connected with the regulation and maintenance of self-esteem-and therefore also with need satisfaction and wish fulfillment (Lampl-de Groot, 1962). What is idealized at each period of the child's development is linked to the source and nature of the injury to the child's narcissism at that period (Kohut, 1966).

The adolescent is in the situation where he experiences the new genital strivings and capacities when his libidinal ties are still to the oedipal and preoedipal objects. The ego experiences this as a danger, and the anxiety and the guilt engendered by this situation become the impelling forces for breaking the tie with the infantile objects. The libido which he withdraws from the infantile object is turned on the ego and the self, resulting in the increased narcissism which so regularly follows upon the breaking of the infantile object ties. It also goes into the idealization of abstractions and moral and ethical values and concepts, for example, asceticism, religious beliefs, philosophies, and intellectuality in general. These idealizations and the new identifications with contemporaries and adults free energies which are neutralized by the ego and in that form are available for aim inhibited pursuits.

This economic formulation accounts for the bursts of sublimations and achievements in adolescence. The stability and the extent of the sublimation also depend on the capacity of the ego to maintain the activity in the conflict free sphere. This may be facilitated when the sublimated activity also serves a defensive function in relation to the drives and the superego. With the stabilization of the ego and with the shift from the narcissistic cathexis of the self of early adolescence to the greater object libidinal cathexis of late adolescence the idealizations and identifications provide the directions for the displacements to aim inhibited goals, and form the basis for choice of work and the mastery of a portion of reality.

For example, the sophomore mentioned earlier remained at the top of his class in college and turned to his work as a haven even at the times of his most acute unhappiness. His family had no intellectual interests and provided no stimulation in this direction during his childhood. Because of his small size he could not fulfill his father's athletic ideals. He was humiliated by his older sister's athletic superiority over him. His intellectual and literary interests started when he idealized a high school English teacher who inspired him and took an interest in his work. Literature and writing also represented something clean, pure, and perfect, in complete contrast to his own dirty, flawed, deteriorating body and his revolting, frank or thinly disguised, incestuous fantasies.

The ego ideal as a structuralized institution of the mind is a development of adolescence. The later stages in the formation of the ego ideal which occur at the end of adolescence illustrate the hierarchical organization and mutual interrelations between ego, ego ideal, and superego, with the ego in the role of active mediator. The adolescent's worldly strivings, his identifications with the realistic images of his parents become aids in the toning down and readjustment of the superego demands, while at the same time the ego calls on the superego for support in restricting the id and in developing mature ego goals and adult achievement standards.

Jacobson (1964) distinguishes between the ego ideal and what she terms the wishful self image, that grandiose, glorified, heroic fantasy figure which may have elements of the ego ideal in the details of its contents, but which is primarily the inflated self image cathected with the libido withdrawn from the infantile object ties at a time when psychological independence from parental objects has not been established and when intolerable anxiety is easily aroused by the hazards of failure if the attempt is made. At the end of adolescence these images tend to become increasingly ego-dystonic, and their persistence beyond their appropriate and useful time precipitates the crises of late adolescence.

One of the main genetic roots of the ego ideal is in the passive feminine homosexual orientation of the negative oedipus complex. In the paper "On Narcissism" Freud (1914) pointed out that it is mainly homosexual libido which is bound in the formation of the ego ideal. This aspect of the ego ideal is very useful in understanding the problems of homosexuality that occur in late adolescence in connection with the approach to the new object and with taking steps in the realistic world which have a crucial quality for the individual in relation to his self-esteem. Conscious homosexual fantasies and episodes of homosexual activity may appear simultaneously with or in alternation with approaches to the heterosexual object. They may have a multiple and shifting meaning in the same individual. They can function as a defense against the fears of being engulfed by the castrated or castrating phallic woman because of the intense passive strivings which arise from the revived preoedipal object ties and the pregenital strivings related to them. They can also represent an identification with the woman in the passive-feminine defense against the oedipal strivings which are stirred up by the approach to the new object. They also appear at times when the main threat is to the vulnerable self-esteem of the adolescent. This especially is the case in those who cling to a grandiose, inflated self image in a compensatory fashion at a time when they are unable to tolerate failure and further narcissistic wounds to an already hard-pressed ego. The threat of failure stems from the pressure to take the steps and make the choices which will define the individual and his place in the community.

At such a point the adolescent may turn to someone who represents his own ideal. The ego is threatened for falling so far short of the narcissistic ideal and the demands of the superego, and is attacked by feelings of guilt and shame. Under these conditions the ego is in desperate need to restore its self-regard. The homosexual libido hitherto bound and neutralized in the ego ideal is reinstinctualized and seeks gratification in the perverse fantasies or activities with the immediately idealized homosexual object, with the idea, "I love and am loved by the kind of person I would like to be." The ego ideal is repersonified in the homosexual object and the process of ego-ideal formation, including the vicissitudes of homosexual libido, may be repeated a number of times. There is also at that point an identification with the idealized qualities of the narcissistic homosexual object.

Two brief clinical vignettes will furnish an illustration. A 19 year-old youth suffered acute anxiety when he was to leave home for college. He dreaded the prospect that he would not be able to make the grade, let alone not live up to his grandiose and inflated expectations. During this period he had a rush of erotic feeling toward two young men each of whom had qualities which he prized and idealized in his grandiose self image.

A 20-year-old youth was constantly "testing himself" for homosexual feelings by monitoring his reactions to older men and contemporaries, to whom he was attracted. At the time he was concerned whether he would be able to establish his potency in a relationship with a girl who was quite hostile and cutting to him at times. Simultaneously, he developed a new friendship with a young man whom he admired. He devoted himself to this relationship with almost equal fervor. At one point he had to fend off erotic feelings toward his friend when they had a long and searching discussion of their relationship with one another while they were sharing the patient's father's bed on a visit to the city. When the immediate issue of potency was resolved for the time being, the friendship cooled considerably. Just as "the evolution of conscience is reproduced regressively [in paranoia]" (Freud, 1914, p. 96), the evolution of the ego ideal may be regressively reproduced in the homosexual attachments of adolescence.

Psychoanalytic Treatment in Adolescence

Psychoanalysts have sounded warnings about the difficulties in the way of psychoanalysis at the height of the adolescent upheaval (e.g., Spiegel, 1961). Anna Freud (1958) gave the most succinct of these when she drew the parallel between the reactions to treatment during unhappy love affairs or periods of mourning and the adolescent's reaction to treatment when his libido is at the point of detaching itself from the parents and cathecting new objects. At such a time the preoccupation is with the present, and little or no libido is available for investment in either the past or the analyst. The later adolescent period, more specifically the college age period, becomes a feasible and even an advantageous time for psychoanalysis. Although he may have been unsuccessful in adequately detaching his libido from the parental objects and still may have no investment in the past, he may make a libidinal investment in the analyst because he seeks relief from his anxiety, depression, and ego-dystonic symptoms. He may also have an increasing awareness that his future love and work life may be threatened. At this time there is normally a change in the ego ideal by which the individual relinquishes the grandiose, heroic, inflated self image for an ideal which can function as a guide to realizable life aims and goals in terms of object choice, career, and role in society. When the ego finds itself in conflict with this ideal and begins to recognize that life goals are threatened and compromised by forces over which the adolescent has no control, he is likely to turn to someone for help. These factors may strengthen the motivation for sustaining the analytic situation and establishing a therapeutic alliance.

Since the older adolescent in crisis who comes to analysis is usually the one who has had a prolonged and difficult struggle over the establishment of his psychological independence from his parents, it is not surprising that this issue and related ones play a central role in the transference, especially in the early part of the analysis. This may take the form of shunning and denying dependence on the analyst as on the parents. At the same time the adolescent tends to regard the analyst as a new and more powerful ally in his search for independence, for the establishment of sexual identity, for finding a new object, and for the definition and~ achievement of life goals. This threatens to heighten the passive, homosexual strivings toward the analyst, to increase the transference resistance in the analysis, and to augment the tendency to act out transference related feelings outside the analysis. The passivity and regressive pull of the analytic situation also contribute to the revival and intensification of the preoedipal object cathexes and the pregenital urges which are connected with them. When these threaten to appear in the transference, they may do so as somatic symptoms involving the autonomic nervous system and may be the initial symptoms of the transference neurosis.

One adolescent described in effect how he split the transference between the transference to the preoedipal infantile object and the transference to the analyst as the guiding, protective father figure, who will watch over his development as a man during this time of instability. He spoke of needing a girl as a break from work, to relax and relieve him, to hold onto and scream at it if he felt like it, whereas the analyst represented "long-term established or establishment help," founded on the assumption that life is really important or significant. As the latter the analyst, by his presence, interest, and attention also functions as an auxiliary ego augmenting the patient's ability to tolerate and recognize infantile strivings without having to resort to action, flight, or immediate gratification so characteristic of adolescence. In this sense analysis tries to ride the wave of progressive stabilization of the ego, which is the normal development of this period and contributes to this stabilization. A consequence for the analysis is a greater tolerance for the appearance and recognition of the transference neurosis and the analysis of it. With these steps the late adolescent shows a greater investment in memory and the past in relation to the conflicts of the present. The analysis loses the quality of merely a communication of current happenings. Analysis of the transference and reconstruction with affective validity become possible.

Analysis provides an opportunity to study the way in which adolescents use drugs in relation to the state of internal conflict, quite apart from their being an established feature of the everyday social scene. Generally, marijuana is used as an institutionalized way of making social contact, and for overcoming inhibitions against them. As observed in the psychoanalytic situation, marijuana and the psychedelic drugs are likely to be used at times of great loneliness, object hunger, narcissistic wounds to the ego, that is, when preoedipal strivings are intensified. The effect of the drug varies with the affective state and the state of ego organization at the time. The existing mood is intensified and reflects the instability of the ego, but the element of seeking for contact with the object is always discernible. Anxiety and loneliness can become a black, empty, frightening despair with the most intense craving for contact with another person. Taking the drug represents an attempt to gratify the wish for relief or reunion with the love object. In this representation the drug taker assumes both roles, the one in need as well as the one who satisfies the need. The recognition that anyone who is "tripping" should have someone with him is not simply a reasonable precaution. For the drug taker it constitutes a valid claim on the immediate interest of another person.

The psychoanalytic situation and psychoanalytic process always have to be considered in relation to the life setting and life circumstances in which they are taking place. From child analysis we know the influence that the developmental level of the child has on indications for analysis, on transference phenomena, and on the motivations for analysis. From training analysis we are familiar with another group of problems linked to the life setting of the analysis. So far as I am aware analysis in the older adolescent age group has been limited almost entirely to college students and those who have dropped out of college. The present-day American college, particularly the residential college, is the major institution provided by our society for the transition from childhood to adulthood where he can find, in Erikson's terms (1956): "a psychosocial moratorium during which extremes of *subjective experience*, alternatives of *ideological choice*, and potentialities of *realistic commitment* can become the subject of social play and joint mastery" (p. 119). This is often a world without work other than academic; limited to a group who are all the same age. The analyst may be the only person outside this age range with whom the youth has any significant human contact for months at a time unless he exerts considerable initiative to do so.

The student status is a mixed blessing for the analysis. At the start it may be a factor in overcoming the fear of passivity and dependence because it can be viewed as another school or college course, like an individual tutorial which meets five times a week. We are prone to assume that the adolescent who comes into an analysis supported by his parents is unequivocally the more passive one. There is clinical evidence to suggest that he may rather be the one who can tolerate this degree of actual dependence without feeling it as a threat to surrender.

With college students there is also the problem of whether the analytic work will be geared to the academic year with its examination periods, long holidays, and frequent interruptions or to a schedule geared more to the needs of the analytic work. If the analyst imposes an immediate intransigent set of conditions, the adolescent may respond as to a parent who forces on him the regressive dependence which still has a strong and dangerous attraction for him and he may be impelled to respond with defiance and flight. On the other hand the analyst may at the start recognize the conflict between the need of continuity in the analytic work and the reality situation of the student who may have no work, no home, no social life, and no community if he stays on for analysis during a long vacation. This approach can enlist the cooperation of the adolescent at the start and leave for later analysis with the analyst with little or nothing else to do, the condition that frequently threatens to intensify the infantile object ties which need to be loosened and relinquished. Adopting this attitude I have found repeatedly that with the progressive analysis of this particular source of resistance the student patient is able to shorten the vacations or remain through them. The normal vacation time is used frequently for significant self-examination without the feeling of being watched, and without the privacy, which is so necessary for adolescents, being intruded upon. The patient frequently returns on a distinctly new level of organization and consolidation.

Summary

Ideally, late adolescence is the time of the last spontaneous developmental consolidation and integration of the personality. In this restructuring of the psychic apparatus the ego gains in power and increases its influence on the id, superego, and ego ideal.

The inevitable moves toward love and work in the realistic world alter the balance between fantasy and reality in the mental life of the individual and make the conditions of pleasure gain more manifest to the adolescent himself. This awareness may become a motivation for treatment. The crises of late adolescence arise when the individual who has not been successful in breaking or loosening oedipal and preoedipal object cathexes is under pressure internally and externally to find a new object and to make self-defining commitments in the realistic world. The reliance of the older adolescent on the new object enables us to study the process by which he makes the transition from the increased narcissistic cathexis of the self so characteristic of earlier adolescence to the object cathexis required for the adult love relationship-a process which is discernible in analysis but which I believe takes place in all male adolescents. In this process the adolescent follows again old pathways from early childhood when the central love object became the stabilizer and organizer for the immature ego.

The formation of an ego ideal that is attuned to reality is a development of late adolescence which is necessary for the adaptive tasks of adult life. The crises of late adolescence are marked by failures of adequate ego-ideal formation and by insufficiently reality-attuned ego ideals which lead to disturbances of sublimation and the capacity for work. Homosexual fantasies and feelings in this age often bring about a fragmentation of the ego ideal as well as regressive efforts to reconstitute it.

The shift of influence to the ego results in anxiety and neurotic symptom formation and increased awareness by the older adolescent that he is in the grip of unconscious forces. This becomes a reliable motivation for entering into and sustaining the psychoanalytic situation.

The life situation of being still dependent on his parents and the setting in which he lives, usually the student status, have an influence on the transference and on technique. But in the neurotic adolescent no basic modification of the analytic situation is necessary.

BIBLIOGRAPHY

Blos, P. (1962), *On Adolescence*. New York: Free Press of Glencoe, Ill.
       (1967), The Second Individuation Process of Adolescence. *Psychoanalytic Study of the Child*, 22: 162-186.
Deutsch, H. (1967), *Selected Problems of Adolescence*. New York: International Universities Press.
Eissler, K. R. (1958), Notes on Problems of Technique in the Psychoanalytic Treatment of Adolescents. *Psychoanalytic Study of the Child*, 13:223-254.
Erikson, E. H. (1956), The Problem of Ego Identity. *J. Amer. Psychoanal. Assn.*, 4:56-121.
Freud, A. (1936), *The Ego and the Mechanisms of Defense*. New York: International Universities Press, rev. ea., 1966.
       (1958), Adolescence. *Psychoanalytic Study of the Child*, 13:255-278.
Freud, S. (1914), On Narcissism. *Standard Edition*, 14:67-102.London: Hogarth Press, 1957.
Geleerd, E. R. (1961), Some Aspects of Ego Vicissitudes in Adolescence. *J. Amer. Psychoanal. Assn.*, 9:394-405.
Jacobson, E. (1964), *The Self and the Object World*. New York: International Universities Press.
Kohut, H. (1966), Forms and Transformations of Narcissism. *J. Amer. Psychoanal. Assn.*, 14:243-272.
Kris, E. (1955), Neutralization and Sublimation. *Psychoanalytic Study of the Child*, 10:30-46.
Lampl-de-Groot, J. (1962), Ego Ideal and Superego. *Psychoanalytic Study of the Child*, 17:48-57.
Pumpian-Mindlin,E. (1965), Omnipotentiality, Youth, and Commitment. *J. Amer. Acad. Child Psychiat.*, 4: 1-18.
Spiegel, L. A. (1961), Disorder and Consolidation in Adolescence. *J. Amer. Psychoanal. Assn.*, 9:406-416.

CHAPTER TWELVE
PSYCHOTIC ADOLESCENTS AND THEIR QUEST FOR GOALS

Rudolf Ekstein

I suggested elsewhere that the frequent turmoil during puberty and adolescence hides a crisis about which it is frequently difficult to decide whether it expresses a sign of growth or is a symptom of pathology, particularly the pathology of schizophrenic and similar psychotic states[7].

Anna Freud in a well-known paragraph from her classic text, *The Ego and the Mechanisms of Defense*, published as early as 1936, has summed up the dilemma with a few master strokes. She describes adolescents as:

> . . . excessively egoistic, regarding themselves as the center of the universe and the sole object of interest, and yet at no time in later life are they capable of so much self-sacrifice and devotion. They form the most passionate love relations, only to break them off as abruptly as they began them. On the one hand they throw themselves enthusiastically into the life of the community and, on the other, they have an overpowering longing for solitude. They oscillate between blind submission to some self-chosen leader and defiant rebellion against any and every authority. They are selfish and materially-minded and at the same time full of lofty idealism. They are esthetic but will suddenly plunge into instinctual indulgence of the most primitive character. At times their behavior to other people is rough and inconsiderate, yet they themselves are extremely touchy. Their moods veer between light-hearted optimism and the blackest pessimism. Sometimes they will work with indefatigable enthusiasm and, at other times, they are sluggish and apathetic[10].

About fifteen years later, Erikson[8] characterized the problem which the adolescent has to solve during this phase of development as the search for a permanent adult role, for occupational, social, religious, and personal commitments which lead him through an identity crisis which is insoluble unless society grants him a psychological and social moratorium This moratorium releases inner organizing forces, enabling the adolescent to move toward young adulthood.

Pumpian-Mindlin[11] has described this phase of the search for commitment, the temporary role diffusion, the playing with and the acting out of future choices, in terms of omnipotentiality, the megalomanic like belief of the adolescent that he can reach any goal while, at the same time, committing himself to nonpermanency. Potentially then, he can reach any goal or none, and during this phase the adaptive or maladaptive struggles of the adolescent will determine the outcome, while he is being watched with anxiety and envy by the parent generation.

Frequently these young people give us distorted pictures of pseudo identification with the adult world. These distortions have been puzzling to the clinician and have encouraged the equally distorted pseudo judgment that adolescence itself is a kind of illness. But it is true that often in this period one can hardly differentiate between psychopathology and normal growth crisis. However, some clear clinical syndromes can be delineated.

In what follows I wish to make remarks about the schizophrenic adolescent whose development parallels in many features that of the average adolescent. His psychopathological state, however, expresses itself in symptoms which, while remindful of the average adolescent crisis, carry in themselves the germs of destructive illness leading to the inability to solve such age-specific problems as the establishment of goals and purposes and the acquisition of skills by which to achieve these goals.

Charlotte Buhler's[2] lifelong studies of the human life cycle and the patterns of establishment of goals, which then, in themselves, become a motivating, organizing, and character-building force, have given us many guidelines. So, too, have Erikson's[9] discussions of the different life stages of man and his studies of ego virtues. These will be helpful as we attempt to throw some light on the schizophrenic adolescent's abortive struggle to develop life goals or *Lebensziele*.

In Charlotte Buhler's terms, the adolescent's attempts at setting life goals are first more experimental and programmatic than realistic. He sees and sometimes tries himself in various roles, but his commitments are temporary. While programming these adult roles, he projects himself in his phantasies into the future. All his moves in relating himself to the future realities of life, however, are provisional and preparatory rather than final. This probing by adolescents is bound up in existential type conflicts. The question "Who am I?" plagues the thinking youth. He feels thrown into conflicts which he cannot resolve and in which he feels utterly alone. Not infrequently his despair leads him to doubt his ability, his wish to cope with life and makes him feel hopeless about himself and sometimes even suicidal.

All these problems occur in an exaggerated form in the case of the pathological development. The neurotic youth may tend either to make premature decisions and enter finite relationships such as a very early marriage or else he may luxuriate in fantasies of future glory and happiness. Thus a borderline schizophrenic and later homosexual girl, Edda, spent her free time at age 12 lying on her bed and dreaming about going to Hollywood with a suitcase full of brilliant plays visiting and charming various famous actors and actresses and becoming famous herself overnight. She prepared maps studied roads to Los Angeles, put money aside, and packed a suitcase with clothes and some of her poems. However it never got beyond that. (Case reported by C. Buhler in preparation.)

The psychotic youths described in the following paragraphs demonstrate four different forms in which their goal setting deviates from the normal, First they have long-range fantasies which as such are phase-characteristic but in their cases are completely unrealistic. Second, in reality they remain "stuck" in short-term goals, which may occur from childhood on or at any age, but which in the psychotic case appear as projects of major proportions. Third, they are unable to integrate themselves and to project a unified self from present to future. And fourth, they experience existential-type conflicts which again although they may be found in normal adolescents in their case become serious struggles involving the question of life or death.

I invite the reader to follow me as I describe some clinical material illustrating these struggles in the psychotherapeutic work with a female schizophrenic adolescent the vicissitudes of whose treatment I have previously described[6].

At first Teresa was hardly reachable and often out of contact. As she slowly ventured out of her autistic world and tried to join the world of her peers as well as that of the adults who were part of her social situation she tried desperately to cope with a catatonic-like paralysis which kept her from putting into action whatever plans she was capable of developing. These plans seemed to remain forever part of her infantile her primitive fantasy world. They reminded one of promises that small children offer their parents in an attempt to secure love but really are not meant to be kept. The difference however between the small child who offers the promise as a love-restoring device and Teresa our patient is that the small child as time passes, learns to deal with the promise in the fullest sense of the word and attempts to live up to it while Teresa's promises could never be kept. They were but static symptoms of her regressed position. They were forgotten as soon as the psychotherapist was out of sight and they could be compared to a repressed dream which one wishes to remember in order to report it to the therapist. When she finally remembered the promise, the mere recollection of it was experienced as if it were the fulfillment of the promise itself. However, as she continued on the slow road to recovery, frequently hardly noticeable, she learned to live up to small promises, which she could now fulfill on the installment plan, as it were.

Her practical life goals that she discussed during this phase of her psychotherapy concerned such issues as being able to leave the shower room not after hours and hours of preoccupation with delusional fantasy activity while under the shower but after a specified time which would permit her to be on time for the volunteer worker who brought her to the clinic for the appointment. Somewhat later she experienced as a major achievement the newly gained capacity to take a bus by herself and to remember the number of the bus. This task occupied her mind for weeks and months until she could triumphantly report that she had reached this goal which she saw as a magnificent achievement, although her performance was completely out of proportion to what would ordinarily be expected of a young person her age.

If one were to see these goals as the life goals she had set for herself one would have to see them as no more and no less than very small very tiny short-term goals. For instance she described during an interview how her social and psychological paralysis finally abated after many weeks and how she was now "moving around a bit, helping the Sisters a bit" in the Catholic home where she then resided. Obviously, this very small investment in the world of reality, the world of social action and of actuality, indicated that much of her psychic energy was invested in other areas of her life. Her life goals therefore were of a different nature than the ones that make up the ambitions, the purposes, the activities of adolescents who belong in the ordinary range of psychopathology or normal behavior.

We will come back to Teresa later. First I want to offer similar material from other patients in order to stress certain interesting aspects of these small short-term goals.

Another research patient was Donald, also a schizophrenic adolescent. He was occupied in establishing his goal behavior with plans for the next few months, such as to be able to eat lunch together with the other children in the private school he attends. It took him months of mastering his anxiety and fear until he was capable of accomplishing this. Other actions concerned his fear of using the public bathroom, of joining children in a baseball game, or of eating and talking together with his parents. He was impelled to discuss these problems for hours and weeks with obsessive rigidity, and one gained the impression that a powerful struggle developed around a seemingly tiny issue.

A third patient, Danny, again an adolescent suffering from an adolescent schizophrenic character disorder, wanted to live up to the promises he thought he owed society and himself and to his ambition to become a musician, a songwriter. These promises to be fulfilled found practical expression in the attempt to finish a poem. He had written the opening lines and was able to complete it only after weeks and months of endless obsessions about it accompanied by escapes into psychotic like acting-out phases. His own enthusiastic response to the finished poem was temporary proof to him that he had a great future but in the face of a minor frustration the enthusiasm vanished without a trace.

What and where are the true investments of such patients The first patient, Theresa, is sometimes capable of establishing a feeble bridge between her inner world, her delusional preoccupation, and her attempts to communicate with the psychotherapist. She does this by means of what I have called *borrowed fantasies*. She can talk about herself only by metaphoric allegories borrowed from television shows or movies to which she is addicted. As she watches these shows she sometimes remembers enough of one so that she can communicate the plot, frequently in a changed and bizarre form and uses the show like a coat hanger on which she hangs her inner life during the transference struggle. The show becomes the brittle and unreliable bridge between her chaotic inner world and the vague desire to talk about that inner world.

During the hour in which she attempted to report to her therapist that she was now successful in "moving around a bit," she used the screen play *Black Orpheus* in order to describe the vicissitudes of the current transference struggle. She saw herself as Eurydice who was involved with Orpheus but who was, at the same time also persecuted by the hateful jealous, and revengeful Aristaeus. She dies a bitter death and Orpheus is to resurrect her. But as he turns around, spurning Pluto's injunction and listens to her desperate pleas, he loses her again. She described, through her powerful identification with the heroine her underlying basic philosophy, which then established the psychotic goal behavior of this patient. She considered herself as dead and at the same time miraculously alive. She lived through and died a thousand deaths and tried to become alive over and over again. She shared with the therapist the powerful and almost convincing fantasy that she was going to kill herself by the end of the year and, at the same time, told him that she has improved so much that she will never touch herself again, blurring the difference between masturbation and suicide. She has gained self-control and she wants to live. But then she projects the very suicidal and/or sexual fantasy into a homicidal or raping expectation, claiming that someone, some man, perhaps some woman, will kill her, attack her, by the end of the year. Her search for love and for acceptance, her struggle against death, are matched at the same time by the search for death. Her fear of death is matched by the fear of life, and like Eurydice, she moves backward and forward between the positions of life and death; and the helper, the beloved one, the rescuer, the therapist, at times is seen as the saviour and at other times as the crucifier, the dangerous murderer, the raper.

One can see then that underneath the conscious, the reality-oriented attempt to master small tasks and to be committed to short-term goals is a powerful psychic system which is characterized by the inner struggle, the alternating commitment to life and to death. One well might say her goal is to stay alive. She does not search for goals which are going to make her life meaningful but rather she struggles for existence itself. The meaning of her life is a life and death struggle.

She finds herself exposed to these powerful anxieties, these inner terrors to such an extent that one well can say of her, if it is permitted to coin a new word, that she does not struggle with omnipotentiality but, rather, that she is beset by omni-impotentiality. She defends herself against the awareness of this omni-impotentiality, this utter helplessness, this terror of dying by means of a defensive fantasy which changes the omni-impotentiality into megalomania. It is for this reason that, in spite of the fact that she does not do more than "move around a bit " learn to take the bus, learn to count money, and so on, she also speaks of goals such as of becoming a famous movie star, an outstanding singer, a great dancer etc. goals that are indeed megalomanic because she can and does do nothing in order to move toward them. They are not goals but fantasies which are to cover up the helplessness, the fear of destruction, the terror of destructive impulses. They are promises to herself by which she tries to restore her self-love and to cope with self- destructive tendencies. These megalomanic fantasy goals are self-promises which are not meant to be kept; they are comparable to the promises of the small child to the parent, and just as the latter promises are made to restore the parent's love these are to restore self-love megalomanic narcissism. They are the psychotic version of what Schlesinger[12] called primary promises.

The same is true of our second patient, Don. He, too even though his accomplishments sometimes move at a snail's pace and are characterized by obsessive repetitiveness which paralyzes him as well as the therapist who attempts to listen, establishes himself in fantasy as a powerful genius a potential world leader, a great pianist one who will impress the world with enormous success. But behind these megalomanic expectations looms large his omni-impotentiality, his utter helplessness and his weakness, his fear of loss of self and loss of object, such as when he tells us that he needs proof that he exists. He sometimes looks at his therapist and wonders whether this experience he has refers to a real person or to a movie-screen picture of the therapist. He must then touch the therapist in order to establish for himself that there is reality. Sometimes he does not believe that he himself exists since he cannot see himself. He would believe that he exists only if he could see his own image and then he needs this evidence to prevent himself from being devoured by anxiety and terror. Descartes' *cogito ergo sum* is replaced by a "you touch me or let me touch you therefore I know that I am and that you are." The third adolescent, Danny, when threatened by loss of object or self-experience or with a kind of psychic death tries to restore object and self-world by destructive acting out through wild aggressive attacks through suicidal gestures of which it is never quite clear if one follows the meaning of the delusional material whether they are to be understood as homicidal or suicidal.

We find then in these patients a variety of common denominators which all relate to the issue at hand: the quasi-search for goals in the psychotic adolescent. As we watch their rudimentary mastery of reality we find that they have endless problems with social adjustment, school learning, work situations, and that they cannot master actuality, that is, apply reality testing to appropriate need-gratifying action. Even in those rare moments when islands of reality testing are comparatively intact, we realize that little energy is available for social mastery, for putting the reality testing into a context of actuality and organized achievement. We notice that small short-term goals dominate their lives as far as realistic problem solutions are concerned. We find also that these patients, within their fantasy activities, see their power, their talents and their gifts, and their possibilities for success way out of proportion to the ordinary daydreams of adolescents. Unlike the successful artists, the writers of whom Freud once said that they achieve through their fantasies what they have dreamed about in their fantasy, namely, honor, power and the love of women, these schizophrenic adolescents have not found the way to translate fantasies or daydreams into truly goal-directed behavior. But still, they see themselves, in spite of evidence to the contrary, as great persons, as world rulers, as creative artists singers, millionaires who must wait for the fantastic fulfillment of their wishes or live with the delusionary conviction that they have reached their goals without ever having to relate these wishes or delusions to any kind of realistic behavior. The primary process does not lead to the secondary process but ends up in a dead-end street. They cannot see any relationship between these fantastic elaborations of their inner dreams and the very small investment they are able to make in their everyday dealing with social issues.

Their megalomanic fantasies however, are not stable, are not constant, and give way frequently not only to underachievement and nonachievement but yield also to terror, to deep-seated anxieties, to the fear of death and annihilation. They fear that they and the world will perish so that most of their inner investment does not constitute a struggle to find meaning in life, to initiate purposeful goal behavior, but rather results in a stay-alive struggle the warding off of *Weltuntergangsphantasien* (fantasies of the world's end).

It must, of course, be emphasized that as these patients struggle for survival and struggle against self-destruction, their use of such existential notions must be understood within the context of schizophrenic thought disorder and disturbed schizophrenic object relations. When we refer to object relations, we do not have in mind the context of interpersonal relations, rather, we refer to the capacity or incapacity of patients to maintain object and self representations within themselves. Theresa, in her use of the theme of Eurydice, gave us a powerful picture of what keeps her from coming to the "upper world", the world of Orpheus and reality, of light and insight, and what keeps her from maintaining this world so that she can establish more than token purposes, more than short-term goals, and can really give meaning to life rather than having to remain committed compulsively to the only meaning she sees in life, the desperate struggle to stay alive to not die. She struggles backward and forward between the attempt to gain the object and to reestablish the self representation and the regression in which she loses both and is paralyzed once more in a catatonic-like disaster.

From studies such as Spitz's[13] we know that the separation and individuation process in the small infant establishes the capacity to maintain self and object representations, an achievement which is then the basis upon which to build realistic goals in life. Adolescents who do not suffer from such weak object and self representation, who are in no danger of really losing them and have resolved this struggle, can move toward purposes in life, can change or maintain these purposes, can develop toward individuation and identity very much along the lines which have been described in the studies of Buhler and Erikson. They sometimes do give the impression that they are about to lose these achievements and, since the adolescent must give up the early objects' ties in the family and replace them with new ties, he lives through phases where these objects and self representations are on shaky ground. But, as we observe such patients during treatment, we see that they go through the ordinary vicissitudes of neurotic transference manifestations and that they utilize the object representation of the analyst in order to bring about reality-oriented life purposes and goals. This the schizophrenic adolescent is unable to do. He therefore develops transferences which are at times only of a neurotic order, but more frequently are actually psychotic transferences in which separation of self and nonself gives way to fusion-states where there is no clear-cut separation between self and object, between therapist and patient. Sometimes these transferences give way to quasi-separations in which either the self or object representation is maintained at the expense of the other. These are then the more autistic like states in which patients seemingly cannot be reached during short phases of the therapeutic process.

We suggest, then, that the inability to maintain goals and goal-directed behavior, the incapacity to establish life purposes which are realistic, stem from the fact that schizophrenic adolescents are unable to maintain object constancy. Unlike their neurotic counterparts who suffer from omnipotentiality, these schizophrenic youngsters suffer from omni-impotentiality, a feeling of impotence which permeates all spheres of life, including the inability to maintain self and object representation. Their defense against this omni-impotentiality, this dread and this hopeless struggle for survival, this constant terror of death, is megalomania, which very frequently looks like the omnipotentiality of the ordinary adolescent but actually is but a forged, a nongenuine replica of it. Since most of their energy, then, must be used in order to reestablish some form of psychic equilibrium, their actual moves seem to be poverty-stricken, slow, token gestures, empty promises, tiny short-term achievements.

Our stress on the issue of object constancy is to indicate the direction in which research in psychotherapy with such patients must proceed. Many case studies[4] in our research help us to establish new techniques utilizable in this struggle toward object constancy. The neurotic adolescent must learn to resolve the unconscious conflict with objects of the past and the present. But still, his is a conflict between separate individuals, between different representations of self, of past and present, and of objects of past and present. The psychotic adolescent offers us a pre-object world and a pre-self world, fused with the partial achievement of object and self representations. As long as there are unstable introjects the purpose and the goal of life will be a desperate and hopeless struggle for existence, a compulsion to endlessly repeat past misery. But when object constancy is achieved, when capacity for object relations is developed such existence will be the basis for new meanings and for permanent and realistic life goals for the release and development of adaptive capacity toward self actualization and the positive use of reality as a source of challenge and nurture[6,14].

References

1. Bugental, J. F. T. Values and Existential Unity, Chapter 22 in C. Buhler and F. Massarik, *The Course of Human Life*, New York: Springer, 1969, pp. 383-392.
2. Buhler, C. *Der menschliche Lebenslauf als psychologisches Problem*, 2nd rev. ed., Gottingen: Verlag fur Psychologie, 1959.
3. Buhler, C. *Intentionality and Self-realization*, San Francisco: Jossey-Bass, inpreparation.
4. Buhler, C. & Goldenberg, H. Structural Aspects of the Individual' s History, Chapter 3 in C. Buhler and F. Massarik, *The Course of Human Life*, New York: Springer, 1968, pp. 54-63.
5. Buhler, C. & Horner, A. J. The Role of Education in the Goal-Setting Process, Chapter 14 in C. Buhler and F. Massarik, *The Course of Human Life*, New York: Springer, 1968, pp. 231-245.
6. Ekstein, R. *Children of Time and Space, of Action and Impulse: Clinical Studies of the Psychoanalytic Treatment of Severely Disturbed Children.* New York: Appleton-Century-Crofts, 1966.
7. Ekstein, R. Turmoil During Puberty and Adolescence: Crisis or Pathology? Reiss-Davis Reporter, 1966, 5:2.
8. Erikson, E.H. *Childhood and Society.* New York: W. W. Norton & Co., Inc., 1950.
9. Erikson, E. H. Reality and Actuality, *J. American Psychoanalytic Association*, 1962, 10, 451.
10. Freud, A. *The Ego and the Mechanisms of Defense.* London: Hogarth Press, 1948.
11. Pumpian- Mindlin, E. Omnipotentiality, Youth, and Commitment, *J. American Academy of Child Psychiatry*, 1965, 4:1, 1-18.
12. Schlesinger, H. J. A Contribution to a Theory of Promising: I: Primary and Secondary Promising. Unpublished, 1964.
13. Spitz, R. A. *The First Year of Life.* New York: International

Universities Press, 1965.
14. Tomlinson, T. The Psychotherapist as a Codeterminant in Client Goal-Setting, Chapter 13 in C. Buhler and F. Massarik, *The Course of Human Life*. New York: Springer, 1968, 212-228.

CHAPTER THIRTEEN
THE BORDERLINE ADOLESCENT:
AN OBJECT RELATIONS VIEW

James Masterson

The clinical syndrome of primary anorexia nervosa has been delineated by Bruch (1962, 1966, 1970, 1971) to consist of a relentless pursuit of thinnest with body-image disturbance of delusional proportions, a deficit in the accurate perception of bodily sensations manifested as lack of awareness of hunger and denial of fatigue, and an all pervasive sense of ineffectiveness. This syndrome is not specific to any one diagnostic category, and debate has continued as to whether a given anorectic patient is schizophrenic, borderline, or psychoneurotic. This chapter attempts to supplement Bruch's work on anorexia nervosa, which stresses interpersonal theory, with my own work on the borderline adolescent and adult, which stresses object relations theory (Masterson 1972, 1974, 1975; Masterson and Rinsley 1975). It will demonstrate how the emphasis in object relations theory (Fairbairn 1952; Guntrip 1969; Jacobson 1964; Kernberg 1971; Klein 1948, 1952; Mahler 1968; Masterson and Rinsley 1975) on intrapsychic structure aids in the clarification of the problem of anorexia nervosa.

A developmental, object relations point of view which goes beyond the symptomatic and descriptive to focus on the development of intrapsychic structures (the differentiation of self and object representations and their related ego defense mechanisms) allows levels of development and types of intrapsychic structures to be distinguished from one another. It is, therefore, a useful tool to distinguish between the various underlying personality structures within which the anorexia nervosa can occur.

Intrapsychic structure develops through the slow, progressive differentiation of the self representation from the object representation and the parallel and related maturation of ego defense mechanisms (Jacobson 1964; Kernberg, 1971). Mahler (1968, 1975) has reported this process as comprising four stages: autistic, symbiotic, separation-individuation, and on the way to object constancy. A developmental failure along this continuum results in an arrest of the differentiation of both the self and object representations and in their related ego functions. The evidence for these arrested structures can then be observed as they are activated, recapitulating the transference. I shall outline three levels of developmental fixation that probably encompass the intrapsychic structure of most anorexia nervosa patients.

If the arrest occurred in the symbiotic phase, the self and object representations would be fused, the patient's ego defenses would be those of the psychotic: splitting, projection, very poor ego boundaries and reality testing, and often delusions and hallucinations. The clinical diagnosis would be schizophrenia.

If the arrest occurred in the separation-individuation phase, the self and object representations would be separate but split into a good and bad object and self representation. The ego defenses would still be primitive but more mature than the psychotic: splitting, clinging, avoidance, denial, projection, acting out. Ego boundaries and reality testing would be weaker than the neurotic but stronger than the psychotic. The clinical diagnosis would be borderline personality organization (Kernberg 1967; Masterson 1972, 1977; Masterson and Rinsley 1975).

If the arrest occurred late in the on-the-way-to-object-constancy phase or in the early phallic-oedipal phase, the self and object representations would be separate and whole rather than split: both good and bad combined rather than being either good or bad. Ego defenses would be more mature with repression supplanting splitting and projection. Denial and acting out would give way to reaction formation or sublimation. The clinical diagnosis would be psychoneurosis.

Most patients with anorexia nervosa probably have a developmental arrest at the symbiotic or separation-individuation phase. Their principle problems evolve around fears of loss of self (engulfment) or loss of the object (abandonment), feelings of emptiness, and struggles over autonomy. The principal problem of those patients with anorexia whose developmental arrest occurred in the fourth phase-on the way to object constancy-would probably revolve around oral pregnancy wishes and fears rather than fears of loss of self or loss of object.

An Object Relations Theory of Anorexia Nervosa

The cause of the developmental arrest in the borderline character appears to be similar to the cause of the arrest in other borderline patients: the mother's withdrawal of her libidinal availability at the child's efforts to separate and individuate. The borderline mother, herself suffering from a borderline syndrome, experiences significant gratification during her child's symbiotic phase. The crisis supervenes at the time of separation-individuation, specifically during the rapprochement subphase, when she finds herself unable to tolerate her toddler's ambivalence, curiosity, and assertiveness, and the mutual cueing and communicative matching essential for the child's individuation fail to develop. The mother is available if the child clings and behaves regressively but withdraws if there is an attempt to separate and individuate. The child needs the mother's supplies in order to grow; if the child grows, however, the supplies are withdrawn. The child's excessive aggression becomes entrenched in consequence of the mother's withdrawal and is further aggravated by the child's inability to integrate positive and negative self and object representations since such integration would require further separation-individuation, which in turn would provoke further withdrawal of maternal libidinal supplies. There thus comes about a situation in which aggression is repetitively provoked without any constructive means conducive to its neutralization.

The images of these two mothers are powerfully introjected by the child to form a split object relations unit which consists of two separate part-units. Each unit consists of a part-self representation, a part-object representation, and an affective component linking the two together. These may be termed the "withdrawing part-unit" and the "rewarding part-unit." The withdrawing part-unit is cathected predominantly with aggressive energy, the rewarding part-unit with libidinal energy, and both remain separated from each other through the mechanism of the splitting defense. The borderline split object relations unit can be summarized as follows:

1. Withdrawing or aggressive part-unit. (a) For part-object representation, a maternal part-object which is attacking, critical, hostile, angry, withdrawing supplies and approval in the face of assertiveness or other efforts toward separation-individuation. (b) For affect, chronic anger, frustration, feeling thwarted, which covers profound underlying abandonment depression. © For part-self representation, a part-self representation of being inadequate, bad, helpless, guilty, ugly, empty, etc.

2. Rewarding or libidinal part-unit. (a) For part-object representation, a maternal pan-object which offers approval, support, and supplies for regressive and clinging behavior. (b) For affect, feeling good, being fed, gratification of the wish for reunion. © For part-self representation, a part self representation of being a good, passive, compliant child.

It is necessary now to inquire into the basis for the persistence of the split ego in these cases. As the child's self-representation begins to differentiate from the object representations of the mother, that is, as the child begins to separate, an abandonment depression is experienced in the wake of the threat of loss or withdrawal of supplies. At the same time, the mother continues to encourage and to reward those aspects of her child's behavior-passivity and regressiveness-which enable her to continue to cling. Thus the mother encourages and rewards in the child the key defense mechanisms of denial of the reality of separation, which in turn allows the persistence of the wish for reunion (clinging), which later emerges as a defense against the abandonment depression. Part of the ego, therefore, fails to undergo the necessary transformation from reliance upon the pleasure principle to reliance upon the reality principle. To do so would mean acceptance of the reality of separation, which would bring on the abandonment depression. The ego structure is now split into a pathological (pleasure) ego and a reality ego, the former pursuing relief from the feeling of abandonment and the latter utilizing the reality principle. The pathological ego denies the reality of the separation which permits the persistence of fantasies of reunion with the mother. Acted out through clinging and regressive behavior, thus defending against the abandonment depression, the patient continues to be able to feel comfortable. Extensive fantasies of reunion are elaborated, projected on to the environment, and acted out, resulting in an increasing denial of reality. The two aspects of the now split ego create an ever-widening chasm between the patient's feelings and the reality of functioning as one gradually moves from the developmental years into adolescence.

The Relationship between the Split Object Relations Unit and the Split Ego

The splitting defense keeps separate the rewarding and the withdrawing object relations part-units, including their associated affects. Both remain conscious but do not influence each other. Although both the rewarding and the withdrawing part-units are pathological, the borderline experiences the rewarding part-unit as increasingly ego-syntonic, as it relieves the feelings of abandonment associated with the withdrawing part-unit. The affective state associated with the rewarding part-unit is that of gratification at being fed, hence, loved. The ensuing denial of reality-the lack of confidence in a self (Bruch's sense of personal ineffectiveness)-seems but a small price to pay for this affective state.

An alliance is now seen to develop between the child's rewarding maternal part-unit and his pathological (pleasure) ego, the primary purpose of which is to promote good feeling and to defend against the feeling of abandonment associated with the withdrawing pan-unit. This powerful alliance funkier promotes the denial of separateness and potentiates the child's acting out of his reunion fantasies. The dramatic clinging behavior of the anorectic performs this function. The alliance has an important secondary function- the discharge of aggression. This is both associated with and directed toward the withdrawing pan-unit by means of symptoms (anorexia), inhibitions of perception of individuative stimuli (i.e., thoughts and feelings), and other kinds of self-destructive acts.

The withdrawing part-unit (part-self representation, part-object representation, and feelings of abandonment) is activated by actual experiences of separation or loss or as a result of the individual's efforts toward separation-individuation within the therapeutic process, which symbolize earlier life experiences which provoked the mother's withdrawal of supplies.

The alliance between the rewarding part-unit and the pathological (pleasure) ego is in turn activated by the resurgence of the withdrawing part-unit. The purpose of this operation is defensive: to restore the wish for reunion in order to relieve the feeling of abandonment. The rewarding part-unit thus becomes the borderline's principal defense against the painful affective state associated with the withdrawing part-unit. In terms of reality, however, both pan-units are pathological; it is as if the patient has but two alternatives- either to feel bad and abandoned (withdrawing part-unit) or to feel good (rewarding part-unit), at the cost of denial of reality and self-destructive behavior.

The Therapeutic Alliance

The patient begins therapy feeling that the behavior motivated by the alliance between her rewarding part-unit and her pathological (pleasure) ego is ego-syntonic: anorexia, clinging, denial of individuation stimuli. She further denies the self-destructiveness of her behavior-the personal sense of ineffectiveness and other reality impairments.

The first objective of the therapist is to render the functioning of this alliance ego alien by means of confrontive clarification of its destructiveness. Insofar as this therapeutic maneuver promotes control of the behavior, the withdrawing part-unit becomes activated, which in turn reactivates the ret warding part-unit with the appearance of funkier resistance. There results a circular process, sequentially including resistance, reality clarification, working through of the feelings of abandonment (withdrawing part-unit), further resistance (rewarding part-unit), and further reality clarification, which leads in turn to further working through. This process of the alternate activation of the two part-units and the defenses of the pathological ego in the transference demonstrates the patient's intrapsychic structure.

In those cases in which the circular working-through process proves successful, an alliance is next seen to develop between the therapist's healthy ego and the patient's embattled reality ego. This therapeutic alliance, formed through the patient's having internalized the therapist as a positive external object who approves of separation-individuation, proceeds to function counter to the alliance between the patient's rewarding part-unit and his pathological (pleasure) ego, battling with the latter, as it were, for ultimate control of the patient's motivations and actions and resulting in structural realignments (Masterson and Rinsley 1975b). In summary, the patient works through the pathological mourning (rage depression) associated with separation from the mother and, through the mechanisms of internalization and identification, eventually forms new intrapsychic structure based on whole object relations.

Clinical Case Illustration

Connie, age fourteen, was admitted to the hospital after a suicidal attempt with a five-year history of anorexia, vomiting, hyperactivity, depression, inability to express her feelings in words, and eventually rage reactions.[1] The illness began at age nine during the summer of her first major trip away from home for a skating competition. She became depressed and escalated her already heavy skating practice schedule. The depression and overactivity continued episodically for the next two years until her eleventh summer when Connie, at camp for the first time, became depressed and began to eat poorly with selective rejection of protein food. During her twelfth year she felt "pressured" in school and was angry with herself when she did not get "the top grades." That year she became terrified at a party when other adolescents began to play a kissing game. She began to cling to her best friend and said she was "turned off" by boys. In her thirteenth year her brother began to withdraw from the family in preparation for his leaving for boarding school the next year and Connie took over many of his household tasks. During the summer she again went away to camp and reexperienced the symptoms of the previous summer, which cleared up on her return.

At fourteen she began to develop breast tissue and an interest in boys, which was accompanied by a ten-pound weight loss. Her mother then developed a severe depression in response to the death of the governess who had raised her, and her older brother left in September for boarding school. Connie became depressed, and by November her selective eating pattern became more noticeable. She was "moody and irritable." By March she vomited regularly, and by April she limited her diet exclusively to vegetables. Attempts by the pediatrician to help were of no avail, and in early September her parents found a suicide note saying she was sorry she was such a burden and describing suicidal attempts by scratching her lower abdomen and attempting to gag herself to death.

Past History

Connie, the second of three children, had a normal birth and early development. She was breast fed until three or four months of age, at which time her mother stopped and reported feeling "a separation, a loss of the feeling of closeness like when Connie was in the womb."

Connie had a succession of nine maids who took care of her. At bedtime Connie often stood in her crib and screamed. Her brother comforted her. Mother said, "There was no point in going on, that would prolong the agony. I was quite upset with guilt feelings." During her first year the mother remembers the patient as a helpful child who never complained, was never a discipline problem, and described her as a clown and mimic who was independent, adventuresome, daring, but obstinate.

Connie was increasingly unhappy during her second year of life when her governess was dismissed. Her mother gave birth to her sister, became depressed, and sent Connie to live for several months with her paternal grandparents. At age four, in nursery school, Connie was settling down after some minor reports of attention-getting behavior when the parents went away for a long weekend and resumed to find Connie "dissolved, depressed, and again anxious about school." Connie was anxious on starting kindergarten to the point that her mother went to school with her each morning for a month. After a tonsillectomy at seven she became "hysterical" and would not let the nurses near her, so her mother took care of her. She did well at school both academically and socially until the last two years. On her mother's prompting the patient took up ice skating at age six, and by age nine was deeply involved in practice and competitions.

Connie's mother was an only child whose mother had died at her birth. She was raised by a governess with whom a strong mutual relationship developed. The governess forced food on her charge and tried to influence her to become a champion ice skater. When Connie's mother was sixteen the governess was dismissed by her father, who had remarried. Mother reacted with a severe depression.

When Connie was born the mother felt consciously that her dream had come true; that her mother had returned in the person of her daughter. The symbiotic themes of reunion, dissolution, fusion. and death that sprang from the mother's relationship with the governess were repeated with Connie, including the problem with food and the ice-skating ambition.

These themes were evidenced in the family sessions when Connie said she no longer wanted to skate. Mother later reported Connie "freezing her out." She said, "I feel so hurt, it's like death. I withdraw." While working through her intense rage and depression at Connie's efforts to separate, she dreamed of Connie's death and of endless empty rooms. She gradually came to see Connie and herself as separate and to support Connie's individuation while looking more realistically at her own life and desires.

Connie's father-a lawyer-was the eldest son of a wealthy, socially powerful family dominated by his mother. He was the "good" son fulfilling all the family expectations. He and his wife continued to live close to and be dominated by the paternal grandmother up to the time of admission. He had a sister, two years younger, who had died at the age of twenty-three of anorexia nervosa. There was evidence of unconscious collusion on the part of Connie's father and the rest of the family in this death. The father named Connie after his sister because "I guess I wanted to resurrect her, to have another chance." It became clear that Connie and this dead sister were fused in the father's mind. In treatment the father began for the first time to mourn the loss of the sister and to explore the formerly repressed feelings of envy, rage, guilt, and sexual desire that he had toward her. He began to see parallels between his interaction with Connie and her symptoms and his past interactions with his sister He reported dreams of trying unsuccessfully to merge two faces (daughter and sister) on one body. Gradually he was able to separate the two, which enabled him to become a father to his daughter.

Intrapsychic Structure

In Connie's intrapsychic structure the rewarding object relations unit consisted of a part-object representation of an omnipotent mother who was perpetually caring and giving her special attention. The part-self representation was of a good child who was loved for behaving as if she were sick, helpless, and could not manage for herself. Affect was of feeling good, a cosmic feeling of safety and protection.

The withdrawing object relations part-unit consisted of a part-object representation of a mother who varied from indifferent to one who was "not there" and "hated her," a part-self representation as "a nobody, evil, fat pig, like I committed ten terrible sins, am ruining the whole family," and an affect of abandonment depression (Masterson 1972).

The defense mechanisms of the pathological ego were denial of separation, splitting, and acting out through clinging to the rewarding object relations part-unit, with a projection on the mother and on others of the wish for reunion. Behavior was helpless, childish, compliant, with avoidance, inhibitions, and denial of individuating thoughts and feelings. This partially accounts for the anorexia, the denial of body image, the helpless self-image. The anger of the withdrawing object relations part-unit was expressed partly by the anorectic symptoms and was partly reflected back on the self as well as projected on those who confronted her acting out of the rewarding object relations part-unit fantasy.

Treatment

Connie was a short, potentially attractive but undernourished, gaunt-looking, depressed girl who weighed sixty-five pounds. She admitted depression but denied the anorexia, weight loss, and hyperactivity. Physical examination was negative, and menarche had not occurred. Her behavior in the hospital was initially hyperactive, overcompliant, and clinging to staff. Her testing was limited to eating, and she used various strategies to conceal from the staff that she was not eating and was vomiting. She denied her cachectic state and hyperactivity and vomited because she was afraid of "getting fat." In interviews during this initial period she related historical data and expressed her sense of helplessness (Bruch's personal ineffectiveness) without her mother and her wish to return to her. Connie's acting out the rewarding part-unit fantasy to defend against the abandonment depression associated with the withdrawing part-unit served the same defensive purpose as the acting out seen in the borderline patient who is openly angry at the mother and whose behavior is destructive (i.e., taking drugs, truancy, etc). The difference between the two is that the latter patient is projecting and acting out the withdrawing part-unit on the mother rather than the rewarding pan-unit. With borderline patients one can frequently find a peer who becomes the recipient of the rewarding part-unit projection.

Limits were set to the patient's acting out by defining a minimum calorie intake per meal; the patient was restricted (i.e., sent to her room for failure to eat the minimum). The feelings associated with not eating then became the subject for the next interview. At the same time her denial and helplessness were confronted.

The confrontation and limit setting triggered the withdrawing part-unit, with increased depression and anger. The withdrawing part-unit was projected on the therapist, and for a long period of time Connie either made angry demands on her therapist, was silent, or attacked him for being stupid and upsetting her. Confrontation of this resistance finally led Connie to confront the withdrawing part-unit and her feelings of abandonment. She said, "There were always so many things I wanted to tell them but couldn't, mostly it was how I felt. I guess I was afraid mother would be angry or get upset. Whenever I told them when I was upset they would get upset too as if I passed it on."

After five months of treatment her doctor's impending vacation triggered the withdrawing part-unit, which Connie acted out with a sign-out letter and loss of weight. When the destructiveness of her acting out was confronted, she turned to transference acting out. She told her therapist, "I did trust you. I don't trust you anymore. You turned against me just when I needed you." Then she continued, "I don't trust my brother anymore either. When he came back from school he acted like he didn't even know me. We weren't even brother and sister anymore. [Sobbing] I had ruined it."

She then returned to transference acting out by acting helpless in the session, which was interpreted as a defense against the previous expressed feelings about being left. In the next session she no longer projected her feelings of being abandoned onto the therapist but continued her examination of the feelings surrounding her brother's departure to school. She then again acted helpless to defend against the anger and depression and again this was confronted. In the next session after some transference acting out she moved further into her dilemma. If she expressed anger at her mother she felt she would be abandoned:

I don't know why, I'm really mad at you. I feel like I could pull your hair out. I'm really mad. I'm scared to death of you more and more. I dread this. When I get mad you just leave. You make me feel like a pea or

something. I've been building all of this inside me. I feel
like I want to take it back, erase it. It's just like at home,
everyone would just leave when I got angry. I'd do things
for my parents so they'd forget I got mad at them.

At this point, in keeping with her style of splitting the anger from
the object and reflecting it back on herself, Connie acted out her helplessness
and hopelessness by a suicide attempt, slashing her wrists which required
stitches. She continued, however, to work through the abandonment
depression:

When I was a little kid they understood and they
showed it, like they loved me in a real way. But as I grew
up they loved me in a fake way, like they didn't know
how. If I grow up and move away, they won't be there
anymore. All my life I've been dreading moving away and
when I think of it I get depressed. All those things-
hugging, kissing- I associated with caring and it was just
the opposite. It's that they cared too much. Normal people
care just by listening. I don't think they care unless they
get down on their hands and knees and hug me. If they
just listen it feels like they're mad. Caring was through
actions and anger was through silence. That makes me
mad to think about that now, that way of controlling me
and I used to be mad at everyone else for not caring
because my parents exaggerated it so. Makes me mad,
makes me furious to think about actions being everything.
I was split inside. It was so difficult to decide when to
appear better and when to appear, worse. It was like they
always wanted me to be happy and I always figured if I
wasn't they'd do things to make me happy. When I was
the worst (helpless) they'd do more things for me, like
love me more. If I wanted to thank them, then I'd make
myself perfect (clinging).

During this twelve-month period of working through, there were
a number of occasions when Connie regressed, stopped eating, and the
eating restriction had to be resumed. These regressions were reactions either
to the depression emerging in the interviews or, on two occasions, to her

doctor's vacation. As she worked through her suicidal depression and homicidal rage a slow, gradual, but drastic change occurred as her individuation began to flower. The clinging behavior stopped, eating restrictions were dropped permanently, depression lifted, she became assertive in interviews, she began to gain weight, and her appearance and dress became much more feminine and appropriate. She then had a series of twelve joint family interviews with her parents, which she managed well. She reported, "I feel good inside because I'm glad about the interviews with my family and feel different about myself I feel different but in a weird way, it's something I have that's mine. I don't feel as afraid of them, that I'm being controlled by them. After I saw them I knew no one told me how to be and I was glad."

She was discharged after sixteen months at a weight of seventy-seven pounds to attend a boarding school and continue in therapy three times a week with her therapist. She did well both at school and in the therapy. Six months after discharge her therapist had to leave, and she has continued with me three times a week for another ten months. She reacted to her therapist's departure with intense regression which seemed limited to her relationship with her mother and to the interviews. She did not become anorectic and continued to do well at school and with her friends. However, she continued to project the withdrawing object relations part-unit onto me and acted out the transference to defend against her feelings of abandonment. Confrontation met only resistance. Perhaps she did not develop symptoms this time because she was discharging the rage in the interviews. Finally, after eight months the transference acting out began to yield to confrontations and she began to work through her feelings of abandonment at her therapist's departure. She reported that she was so hurt and angry at his leaving her that she vowed to never allow a relationship like that to develop again. Thus, after thirty two months of intensive psychotherapy she had made good progress but still had much to accomplish.

Discussion

Bruch's interpersonal theory postulates that anorexia nervosa is due to a rigid effort to control the body in order to establish a "domain of selfhood" when faced with the adolescent growth task of independence and identity formation. Object relations theory postulates that anorexia nervosa has a number of adaptive and defensive purposes. Its intrapsychic defensive purpose is to relieve anxiety about loss of the object during separation and individuation by avoiding growth of all kinds-physical, sexual, emotional-and to discharge the tension associated with hostility to the object. Its adaptive purpose is to provoke the mother's attention at the same time hostility is expressed toward the mother. The anorectic symptom is the keystone to a whole set of pathologic defenses whose purpose is to preserve the object at the cost of the self-the latter being denied. Confrontation of this denial in the therapeutic relationship leads to a working through of the depression and rage at loss of the object and allows separation-individuation to resume. The key difference between the two theories is that object relations theory links the symptoms with the self, the object, the affective state, and the defensive mechanism, that is, the whole underlying problem in intrapsychic structure.

Bruch's evidence for a failure to learn body perceptions is very persuasive. There is, however, much evidence to suggest that the borderline patient suppresses and denies those individuating thoughts, feelings, actions, and, possibly, perceptions that might interfere with the wish for supplies from the mother.

Bruch describes a sense of personal ineffectiveness related to always acting in response to others. Object relations theory suggests that helplessness (a common symptom in the borderline) is an inevitable consequence of separation-individuation failure and clinging. The predominant affect is invested in the object, not the self. Since efforts at coping and mastery are met by fear of loss of the object, the patient avoids efforts to cope and consequently feels helpless to cope on her own.

Bruch further describes the patient not relying on her own thoughts, feelings, and body sensations as manifesting a defect in initiative. Object relations theory suggests that this lack of autonomy, like helplessness, is again a consequence of separation-individuation problems-the patient denies and suppresses individuation to preserve maternal supplies.

Bruch describes "an unrelenting No" extending to every area of living and aggressive negativism against all therapy. Object relations theory suggests that the "No" represents an expression of rage at the demand that the self be given up to obtain supplies; this rage is projected on all expectations and expressed by opposition. The negativism to psychotherapy is more specific. Psychotherapy symbolizes separation-individuation and as such triggers the withdrawing object relations part-unit which is projected on the psychotherapy which is then resisted.

While Bruch describes the parents of anorectics as "appearing" normal, they superimpose their needs on their children, disregarding signals, and the children lack appropriate confirming responses. We have not found the first point to be true, and the second point, while true, requires substantial elaboration. None of our parents, including the parents of patients with anorexia nervosa, ever appeared normal. Both parents were usually clinically ill; the mother usually borderline and the father either borderline or manifesting a character disorder. The mother clung to the patient to relieve her own anxiety. She did respond to and confirm the child's clinging behavior but did not confirm individuating behavior. The father distanced himself from the patient while, at the same time, reinforcing the mother's clinging. The patient's regressive behavior played a vital role in maintaining the mother's equilibrium and often was the basis of the family's system of emotional relationships leading to a depersonification (Masterson 1972; Rinsley 1971).

The past history of the child is described by Bruch as being apparently normal with excellent performance and free of any difficulties. Object relations theory would assert that this very performance based on the clinging mechanism is most pathologic because it serves to avoid individuation. In addition, many of our patients had symptomatic episodes in their childhoods.

Bruch suggests adolescence itself as a precipitating event along with new experiences such as going to camp or entering a new school or college. Object relations theory is of specific use here since it not only suggests what events are important but also indicates why. Any environmental event that threatens the relationship with the person to whom the patient is clinging (i.e., death, divorce, depression, etc.) exposes the youth to separation anxiety and abandonment depression. Similarly, any event which poses a challenge that requires individuating coping (i.e., new school, camp, college, etc.) interrupts the patient's defense mechanisms and exposes the adolescent to separation anxiety. Many events combine both factors.

The need for independence and identity that arises in adolescence, Bruch suggests, precipitates the condition. Although these factors may play a role, object relations theory makes clear that it is a precipitating factor only to the degree that it stirs up earlier separation-individuation problems and brings on separation anxiety and abandonment depression. Bruch states that the underlying structure of the disorder is not specific but resembles other disorders of adolescence. It is true that the symptom complex itself is not specific, but the underlying structure-be it borderline, schizophrenic, or psychoneurotic-is quite specific and should be so diagnosed for effective therapy.

With the phrase "the constructive use of ignorance" Bruch stresses the need to evoke awareness of impulses, feelings, and needs originating within the patient by the therapist's confirming or correcting responses to the patient's self-initiated expressions. I agree with this approach on the basis that its objective is to help the patient separate and individuate. There is, however, one important exception in the initial phase of psychotherapy. The patient's denial of the destructiveness of the rewarding object relations part-unit pathologic ego alliance to individuation is unconscious, and the anorectic cannot initiate the processes necessary to overcome it alone. The therapist must aid the patient by questioning and confronting the denial. An independent self-motivated desire for therapy emerges as the patient becomes aware on the one hand of individuating thoughts and feelings and on the other of how the behavior has been destructive to this essential image of the self. Transference distortions produced by this activity must be taken up later in psychotherapy as the patient becomes aware of the contrast between individuation strivings and clinging transference.

Conclusions

In my view, the advantages to supplementing Bruch's interpersonal theory with this object relations theory are that it completes the puzzle of the clinical picture by providing the missing intrapsychic piece. Tying clinical manifestations to their developmental roots provides a more comprehensible and clearer picture of the disorder as a whole which then allows for the design of a more accurate psychotherapy. This approach clearly emphasizes, as well as explains why, the objective of psychotherapy of anorexia nervosa should go beyond weight gain to emotional growth-the patient's only guarantee against the future.

NOTES

I am indebted to Bruce Bienenstock, M.D., for the material summarized here.

1. The parents each received individual psychotherapy and group therapy once a week for sixteen months. I am indebted to Mrs. Grace Christ, M.S.W.. the parents' therapist, for the material summarized here.

References

Bruch, H. 1962. Perceptual and conceptual disturbances in anorexia nervosa. *Psychosomatic Medicine* 24: 187- 194.

Bruch, H. 1966. Anorexia nervosa and its differential diagnosis. *Journal Nervous and Mental Diseases*, 141:555-565.

Bruch, H. 1970. Psychotherapy in primary anorexia nervosa. *Journal of Nervous and Mental Diseases*, 150:51-66.

Bruch, H. 1971. Death in anorexia nervosa. *Psychosomatic Medicine*, 33: 135- 144.

Fairbairn, W. R. D. 1952. *Psychoanalytic Studies of the Personality.* London: Tavistock.

Guntrip, H. 1969. *Schizoid Phenomena Object Relations and the Self.* New York: International Universities Press.

Jacobson, E. 1964. *The Self and the Object World.* New York:International Universities Press.

Kernberg, O. F. 1967. Borderline personality organization. *Journal of the American Psychoanalytic Association*, 15:641-685.

Kernberg, O. F. 1971. New developments in psychoanalytic object relations theory. Paper read to the American Psychoanalytic Association, May 1971, Washington, D.C.

Klein, M. 1948. Mourning and its relation to manic depressive states. In *Contributions to Psychoanalysis* (1921-1945). London: Hogarth.

Klein, M. 1952. Notes on some schizoid mechanisms. In J. Riviere, ed. *Developments in Psychoanalysis.* London: Hogarth.

Mahler, M. S. 1968. *On Human Symbiosis and the Vicissitudes of Individuation.* Vol. 1. New York: International Universities Press.

Mahler, M. S. 1975. *The Psychological Birth of the Human Infant.* New York: Basic.

Masterson, J. F. 1972. *Treatment of the Borderline Adolescent: A Developmental Approach.* New York: Wiley.

Masterson, J. F. 1974. Intensive psychotherapy of the borderline adolescent with a borderline syndrome. In *American Handbook of Psychiatry.* Vol. 2. New York: Basic.

Masterson, J. F. 1975. The splitting defense mechanism of the borderline adolescent. In I. E. Mack, ed. *Borderline States.* New York: Grune & Stratton.

Masterson, I. F. 1977. *Psychotherapy of the Borderline Adult.* New York: Brunner/Mazel.

Masterson, J. F., and Rinsley, D. B. 1975. The role of the mother in the genesis and psychic structure of the borderline personality. *International Journal of Psychoanalysis*, 56:163-177.

Rinsley, D. B. 1971. The adolescent inpatient: patterns of depersonification. *Psychoanalytic Quarterly*, 45:3-22.

CHAPTER FOURTEEN
FAMILY TRANSACTIONS IN THE ETIOLOGY OF DROPPING OUT OF COLLEGE *

Edgar Levenson, Nathan Stockhamer and Arthur Feiner

During October 1966 *The New Yorker* magazine ran a very funny cartoon by Saxon, showing the entrance hall of a rather elaborate town house. A door in the rear opens onto a neatly tended garden. The wife is standing on the stairs, one hand clutching the balustrade, looking apprehensive. Her white-faced husband, nattily attired in a madras dinner jacket, is talking earnestly into the telephone. The caption reads: "Listen to me, Francine *Stay* in Wellesley! We can discuss who you are and who I am over the vacation!"**

This cartoon captures, as no words can, the sudden shock experienced by these conventional and rather complacent parents as they make their first contact with the language of adolescent identity crisis. For many hapless parents, no amount of telephone coaching imploring, or bribing will prevent their children from joining the ranks of the dropouts, for over 50 per cent of the million students entering college across the country leave before completing the regular course of studies.

Now this is, we must confess, an alarmist statistic. Many students return after an interval to the same or another college. Many do quite well without ever going back. Many never belonged or wanted to be in college in the first place. But, even when these categories are eliminated from consideration, one is still confronted with a very large part of the dropout population whose defection is accompanied by serious emotional disability, much misery and psychological hardship, and sometimes even when these youngsters return to college, a "burned-out" adjustment without gusto or productivity.**

We have maintained at the William Alanson White Institute of Psychiatry,

*Presented in a slightly different from by the senior author, (Edgar A. Levenson) at the December 1966 meeting of the William Alanson White Psychoanalytic Psychology. The authors are indebted to all the members of the Institute's College Dropout Project who have contributed to these formulations, particularly to Dr. Martin Kohn for his data collecting designs, Mrs. Ruth Tendler and Mrs. Majorie Newstrand for their intake screening, and to all the therapists for their clinical and theoretical insights.
Aided by grant OM-867, National Institute of Mental Health.
**The New Yorker, October 15, 1966.

Psychoanalysis and Psychology a clinic for the treatment of college dropouts which has been in continuous operation for the past five years. We intend in this paper to describe our experience with this group, which represents only a selected and not entirely representative sample of the dropout population, our patients were all referred by the colleagues or, as our reputation grew, self-referred. Since they followed through on the application procedure with its voluminous questionnaires and inevitable delays, we may assume they were motivated or, at the very least, persistent. There are certainly large categories of dropouts we never see. For example, we tend not to see the casual dropout who takes a year off to travel, the grossly inept dropout, the motivated dropout who joins the Peace Corps, the student who leaves school to get married, to start his own business, or to enter a career in the Arts. Nor do we see many of the emotionally distressed dropouts who evade the screening college counselors by offering some version of the above reasons.

One might question extrapolating from our group to the dropout population at large, or even the emotionally distressed dropout group. However, studies by Murphey, Silber, et al.[23] of so-called normal families, Keniston of alienated students[11] and Yale dropouts,[12] and the observations of other investigators,[25] seem to substantiate many of our clinical impressions. Obviously further comparison studies, on campus, will be required to validate our hypotheses.

What we do see are students characterized by *inaction*, almost really *non-action*, inasmuch as it appears to be more determination not to act than indifference. These students drop out of school and drop out of society. They return home, do nothing, frequently sleep all day, go out at night, constitute a loyal component of the late-late show audience. If they do leave home, they join marginal beat groups, living in a kind of non-action commune. This group should be of interest to psychoanalytic audience, not just because there are so many of them, but because they manifest a clinical syndrome we are seeing with increasing frequency, not only in adolescents but older patients as well. Dropping out is becoming a signature of the times; not only from college, but marriage, parenthood, job-all the socially defined and validated roles expected of competent adults. We are seeing, increasingly, people who have demonstrated the ability to perform, often very well, and then stop. This is certainly true of the dropout who had previously manifested sufficient school competence to carry him into college.

---

* According to Dana Farnsworth, at Harvard, more then 50 percent of the total dropout population have a significant emotional component in their difficulties.[8]

In other words, people who have demonstrated previous sexual, work, and social competence refuse to or are unable to couple their demonstrated competence to the appropriate social role. All symptoms may be considered a choice of action, however out of awareness. And, if action is considered to lie on a continuum, then patients are moving increasingly from the action directed inward (the autoplastic mode) to the action directed outward (the alloplastic mode). The hysteric says, "I'd love to perform, but I can't, I'm paralyzed." The obsessional says, "I can and do perform, but it is out of a sense of duty. I get no pleasure from it." And, now we are hearing a new refrain," "Well, I can perform and I have, but I don't want to." I do not mean to imply that those in this last category experience neither anxiety nor guilt; but, unlike the conscientious obsessional who performs in spite of distress, these people take refuge in inaction, or, at least, inaction in the conventional social roles. We would like to label this behavior *sociopathy*, limiting that term to its most literal sense; to wit, pathology in the area of social functioning.*

Our thesis is that dropping out may not be simply a random event in the lives of a heterogenous group of people, but rather a significant parameter of behavior; important enough to justify defining a group by its presence and labeling the behavior sociopathic. In describing our population, we hope to suggest how this syndrome can develop, and some of the problems in treating it. We must point out that we started this project with much more limited directions than we now have. Interest in dropouts arose out of the pre-existing Young Adult Treatment Service, which had accumulated some three years of experience. Both at this service and in our own practices, we had noticed an increasing number of college dropouts. As was indicated in our opening paragraph, the attrition rate is astonishing. Psychotherapists working on the college campuses felt that, as a group, these students were most difficult to identify and treat. There was some feeling that they might require the dropping out as a commitment to, at least, failure before they would even consider counseling or therapy. Also, they often believed, and with some justification, that the college clinic was regarded as part of the establishment of the university, the secular arm so to speak, and therefore untrustworthy.

We had some feeling that a community facility, off the college campuses and separate from the college establishment, would be more likely to draw these students; and would give us an opportunity to have a concentrated population for study and to see what the effects of psychotherapy would be and whether they would stay in the Clinic.

As a consequence, in 1962, we obtained from the National Institute of Mental Health a grant for the limited design of establishing a small clinical facility. This was not, in any sense, a research project and we had no feeling at that time that we were dealing with, in any sense, a homogeneous population. We had developed and implemented a whole series of data collecting forms and questionnaires, which we had intended really only to collect demographic data about the student and their families.[13] We were trying more to develop the forms and structure of a clinic rather than to collect specific data. The statistics and findings of the clinic have been presented in a variety of journals and as a chapter in a recent symposium.[4,13,14,16-20]

There is, of course, a great deal one can say about variations of the dropout syndrome. Girls are different from boys. Students who drop out in the first year are different from students who drop out in the senior year. Those who finish the term and then leave are different from those who leave in mid-semester. Some students sit about and passively fail-waiting to be thrown out. Some act out, act in "trouble." Some call their parents to take them home, or become ill. Some make suicide attempts, a few become psychotic. Commuter college students (living at home) are different from live-away students. Some leave in excellent scholastic standing. The diagnostic categories range from passive character disorder to schizophrenia (oddly enough with severity of diagnosis increasing with each year of college). In other words, when we attempted to classify the students, we found we had a pastiche of diagnoses and behavior patterns. Moreover, everyone seems to agree that anything one can say of the dropout can be said with equal conviction of students who stay in school. No test pattern, diagnostic category, or pattern of study habits clearly differentiates dropout from stay-in. Why does one severe obsessive student with homosexual pre-occupations stay in and be thrown out. Some act out, act in "trouble." Some call their parents to take them home, or become ill. Some make suicide attempts, a few become psychotic. Commuter college students (living at home) are different from live-away students. Some leave in excellent scholastic standing. The diagnostic categories range from passive character disorder to schizophrenia (oddly enough with severity of diagnosis increasing with each year of college). In other words, when we attempted to classify the students, we found we had a pastiche of diagnoses and behavior patterns. Moreover, everyone seems to agree that anything one can say of the dropout can be said with equal conviction of students who stay in school. No test pattern, diagnostic category, or pattern of study habits clearly differentiates dropout from stay-in. Why does one severe obsessive student with homosexual pre-occupations stay in and function and another drop out?

Although there are now a number of long-term follow-up studies of college dropouts,[24] there have been no effective efforts at correlating nosology with eventual prognosis for return to school. Indeed sometimes those students considered diagnostically "sickest" return and sustain brilliant scholastic careers, while mild "passive-dependent" types languish for years. About all that can be said and that impressionistically, is that there seems to be an association between the quality of the student's functioning at the time of his departure and the rapidity of his return to acceptable performance. Those students who leave in good scholastic standing, whether they have finished the term or not, might be said to have shown more initiative shall those students who let the school situation die under them. As one might expect, the prognosis for quick and successful return seems better for the former group.

In the first five years of the project we screened 235 students, and started 90 in treatment. We saw them once a week, started two group therapy projects and somewhat later, really under pressure from the parents for help, we initiated a parent discussion group. We held a weekly one and a half-hour staff conference, intended for a discussion of treatment problems, but which shortly became a textbook example of violent peer group countertransference. These experiences and their meaningfulness have been eloquently described elsewhere by Akeret and Stockhamer.[4] Rather than concluding, as we had first suspected, that our difficulties in being helpful to each other were caused by ineluctable personal shortcomings (in each other, naturally) we began to suspect that it might have something to do with the nature of our patients.

It was at this point, we believe, that the project really came alive. We probed our reactions to the students. First, they evoked a good deal of anxiety in us, more shall one might attribute to the pressure to "reach" them, to understand them. We felt, all of us, dreadfully "square" and intimidated by their scorn. We were impressed by their unconventionality and daring to fail. Finally, we suspected we were secretly intrigued by their defiance. Were they doing what we did not dare to do? And were not their lives often rather colorful? Some of them took drugs, went on "acid" trips, had unconventional sexual experiences. Were we jealous? Somehow we seemed to feel like terrible fakes. Seen through their eyes, one virtually reeked of hypocrisy, cant, and banality. No wonder we attacked each other. As Akeret and Stockhamer have indicated, each therapist, in presenting a case, hoped-to his eventual disappointment and despair- that the group would support and reassure him.[4]

To inquire into this aspect of our reactions to the patients and to each other, we questionnaired ourselves about our own school histories, dropouts-abortive and real, and so on. Slowly we became more insightful-and humble. Indeed, we began to get much better. Unfortunately, however, the patients continued quite unabashedly in their non-performance. It occurred to us then that somehow we were in the same boat as the parents. We would say to ourselves, "What have we done wrong? Where have we failed? This was actually a narcissistic inquiry, meaning, "Why don't they do what we want?" Or-echo of the parents-we would say, "The trouble with these kids is...."

It seemed quite reasonable to assume that if one understood the patient's experience with his family, who they were and how they behavior, it would be considerably easier for us to discover what roles we were haplessly recreating. From the very beginning, we strongly felt *not only* that the students projected onto us distortions from their past experiences, but that they were able to call out in us intense irrational participations which recapitulated their earlier experience. In short, they had a remarkable ability to recreate with new persons their previous environment: "To make themselves at home." This is a quality worth noting, since it can be correlated with specifics of the family experience, and helps explain how these students in a variety of campus settings could so strikingly re-experience the destructive ambience of their family lives.

We reviewed more carefully our data on the families and began to interview and offer treatment in a group(s) to the parents. One statistic relevant to the parent population seemed important. At first, we had suspected it might be an artifact, but it appeared with considerable regularity in our private practices, and colleagues on the campuses had also noted it. A very high percentage of the parents had some interruption in their own schooling. Many of them had left school either in high school or college. Some of them had completed college or even graduate training and then not used it. For instance, we had several parents who had earned law degrees and were then functioning in a relatively marginal or unchallenging occupation. In our first year, 68 per cent of the fathers and 61 per cent of the mothers had interruptions in their schooling. Many of them had been in college during the depression and had to leave for financial reasons. A startling number were older children who had left school for financial reasons, and had returned home to become the supports of their families while a younger child went on to college successfully.

In addition to the interruptions in schooling, one-third of our population had an interruption in family life-that is, came from broken homes. In over half of the broken families, there had been separation, often for years, without a final divorce; that is, they did not incisively break up and go on to a new life. If one groups the following factors: parents' severe disappointments in their careers, scholastic interruptions, openly expressed mental disorder, discontinuity in family experience (death, divorce, desertion), one or more of these factors were true in over 85 per cent of our patients. It could have been artifactitious, but it also pointed a way in which the parents might have a complex investment in their children's performance. Again, with Kohn's questionnaire designs, we began to assess such factors as the parents' ambition for the child as well as their degree of constructive support and implementation.[13] We found, as one might expect, that the parents tended to be quite ambitious, the mothers even more so than the fathers. At the same time the degree of valid constructive support given their children was remarkably low. We also found some consistent patterns of child rearing, particularly in attitudes concerning toilet training, privacy, and infantile sexual behavior.

Ruth Tendler and Joannne Levenson, who were interviewing and studying the parents, were struck by the degree in which these parents do not see their children as separate; that is, the mothers act as if the child never did *anything* that they did not know about.[21] They were struck by a consistent finding of a lack of any real rebelliousness in early infancy, childhood or adolescence. These children had been toilet-trained easily, had slept well, had always done what they were told. They were, in a word, model, well-behaved "good children," rarely if ever openly rebellious or difficult, despite a great deal of pressuring and interference from the parents. These were families with a high incidence of relatively inadequate personal and social performance, very involved with their children, ambitious for them, yet unable to present first-rate models for identity and growth. A recurring family pattern would show a dissatisfied, seductive mother, holding her husband in disesteem. He is, in turn, both invested in his child's success to prove that he has produced something of worth, and, yet, in a subliminal competition for the respect and attention of his wife.

This is very much the family constellation described by Keniston[11] for his uncommitted students; by Lidz, Fleck, et al. for families of schizophrenics; Bieber[5] for homosexuals, and Erikson[7] for identity crisis. In a word, it is the ultimate psychoanalytic banality, explaining everything from schizophrenia to ingrown toenails. Kenniston quite properly asks how can one distinguish the preconditions for these states if the family structure seems so similar.*

In other words, the *specificity of symptom choice* depends considerably on the family style; on what is permitted and what is not. It does not depend as much on the frustration of basic needs or universal dynamisms. For example, many of these students suffer severe maternal deprivation; the lack of mothering and the consequent distrust, depression and dependent clinging is certainly the *vis a tergo* for many dropouts. Yet, it is the particular balance of the family system, its values and rules, which make it possible for the student to drop out rather than remain as a compulsive student, develop migraine or a depression, or commit suicide.

There is an increasing feeling, then, among investigators that family dynamics supply a clue to the specificity of symptom choice. We are not suggesting that family experience is an absolute determinant of subsequent behavior. It is, however the *anlage* for dropout performance. Whether the dropout actually occurs depends on a variety of factors, such as the climate of the college, influence of peers, sexual difficulties, military status, influence of teachers, and so forth. There is much the colleges can do to influence the dropout's decision, positively or negatively. Ford at Penn State has inaugurated a rather elaborate program geared to minimizing situational maladjustments and misplacements, with considerable success.[10] It will be evident that to the extent that the colleges can avoid inadvertently recapitulating the family dynamics will be all to the good. To the extent that the college, *in loco parentis*, reinforces the neurotic operations of the family, a collapse becomes more likely.

Now, what are (a) the family dynamics and (b) the family ethology which produced the dropout? Family dynamics encompasses a concept in which the symptomatology of the "designated" patient is revealed to be only a facet of a multiperson family disturbance. The symptom of the patient balances intrafamilial forces as well as intrapsychic forces. The family is seen as a complex interlocking homeostatic system wherein the intrapsychic struggles of the members meld into a transactional whole. We use the term *family ethology* to distinguish the pervasive flavor and style of the family as a subcultural group from the characteristics of the group as a homeostatic system.

We would like first to present what we consider the three cardinal characteristics of the families we have seen and which have, we think, much to do with our growing conviction that failure is destiny in these families. Then we would like to discuss briefly some of the specific checks and balances which occur within the family system. These three ethological characteristics are *(1) unautheniticity; (2) disenchantment; (3) incipient rebelliousness.*

1. *Unauthenticity*: There is a very strong tone of fakery about these families. Despite their unhappiness, joylessness and disappointment, often in denial of very disturbed marital relationships, they maintain for the child and the outside world a powerful fictional image of the good family without difficulty or friction, this "pseudo-mutuality" requires that here be no criticism of each other by parents and children. When there is friction or personal distress it is quickly forgotten, denied, or minimized. The family fiction is that they have always "gotten along well" together. The children were raised according "to the book," whatever the current vogue was, Watsonian behaviorism, Spock, and so on). When the book clanged, the parents changed too.

2. *Disenchantment*: Although they are very hard working and industrious, they are people who experience very little pleasure and live with very little gusto. Although financial and career dissatisfactions lie close to the surface, there seems in addition a profound life-time low grade depression, much self-deprivation, and denied anger. They hardly give the child much sense of the rewards of adulthood; rather, he is pressured to be successful so that he will be able to carry the burden of adult life. They do not say encouragingly, "Finish college, grow up so that you can enjoy work, marriage, life." Rather they admonish, "Hurry up, grow up, get strong before you're smashed by the juggernaut."

3. *Incipient Rebelliousness*: This is the most interesting aspect of this tangled web of motivations. Many of the parents had periods of rebelliousness in their early adulthood. They had been political rebels, had tried careers in art or music or the theater, had married women their families disapproved of, attempted audacious business undertakings, then collapsed and returned to security, to civil service, to family businesses, to pedestrian jobs. Still, almost none of our parents is a "company man." None of them works for a large paternalistic corporation. They are, in a sense, bohemians

manques.

Their rebelliousness and dissatisfaction would not, per se, make trouble for the child. It might even encourage him to break away, to complete more successfully his parents' incipient rebellion. The child might, in Singer's terms, develop his own identity without pathological identification with the parents' failure.[27] The unauthenticity however requires that the rebellion and dissatisfaction be denied. Without the appearance of well-being, the "good parent" image would collapse and the self-esteem of the parents would be shattered. Consequently, the child comes to play an important role in the family homeostasis. Here, Ackerman's four postulates are appropriate: (1) How does the behavior of the child serve as a symptom of the emotional warp of the family; (2) how does it reflect an urge to heal what ails the family; (3) how does it serve as a stabilizer of a pre-existing family equilibrium; and (4) how does it symbolize the growth potential both of the individual and the family.[1,2,3]

One could extrapolate the answers from what we have already related about the families. One of us has presented the homeostatic aspect in detail elsewhere,[16] but briefly we would like to elaborate on the third postulate.

We see the failure of the student playing an important homeostatic role for the family. Successful individuation actually threatens the family integrity. We have seen previously bland marriages explode and break up when the students go away. Parents often come shockingly into contact with the aridity and disappointment of their lives when the child leaves home. Students are often cued in by telephone calls and letters to come home. This is not dissimilar from the experience of the young child who goes off to camp and develops the panicky belief that something might happen to his parents if he is not there. But we wish to emphasize that it is not without reality. Sometimes, when the family scapegoat begins to improve in college; one of the other previously impeccable siblings folds up. In short, dropping out often seems to meet Ackerman's criteria for a family homeostatic operation.[1] This is not to imply that the scapegoat is nothing more than the passive victim of his family. The rewards of being the family victim are great. One is also the family savior. The secondary gains are considerable and the victim, as the therapist soon comes to realize, resists being lifted from his altar.

To summarize, the most striking *desideratum* of these families is to maintain the air of pseudo-mutuality. Unlike a schizophrenic family, this is not managed by tolerating or encouraging bizarre behavior, but rather by insisting on normalcy, within the family. They might be compared to a member of a tribal group, a Navajo or Apache, who has no difficulty while he stays on the reservation but runs into great trouble when he enters the general community. That is to say, unlike the schizophrenic or the acting-out child, these people seem to have relatively little difficulty as long as *they stay together*. Their largest trouble seems to develop when one member of the group moves out.

This odd tribal integrity in the family fitted in with some observations that Joanne Levenson had made in studying the cultural patterning of the families.[21] What was evident in her study was the stylistic ethnocentricity of these family groups. For instance, many of them had a network of three-generation closeness; that is, the parents in close proximity to their own parents, often living in the same neighborhood or even living in the same house. Many of our students had been taken care of a great deal or had early nurturing experiences with the grandparents. These were families which were also ethnocentric in the sense that they had relatively few friends and those were strikingly similar to themselves. They were in terms of their mores and values very parochial and highly insular. Even when they were intellectually advanced and cultivated esthetically, they were not at all open to styles of life that were different from their own. Joanne Levenson postulated, we believe correctly, that one of the real difficulties for these families is the marked discontinuity between the family culture and the general culture into which the student must emerge.

In other words, another way of looking at the difficulties these families have is to examine in addition to the intrafamilial dynamics, what happens when a potential dropout family as a relatively stable self-perpetuating system with its own *ethos* comes into contact with the larger societal system. It is at this *tribal interface* that the symptomatology of the dropout student becomes quite evident. As in a primitive tribal group, where there is a high survival priority on getting along together, one tends to direct aberrant behavior to the outside. Thus, one may not get angry with one's father; one decides that he is being bewitched by an outsider. It is of parenthetic interest that studies of children with early school phobia note that the parents tend to defend the children against the school, holding the establishment responsible for the child's difficulties. Thus, in addition to the unauthenticity and the powerful pressures to maintain tribal appearances, these families give tacit support to the some what paranoid position-"Blame them, don't blame us!" This may be partly the basis of student complaints about the schools. One hears this often rationalized by students into protests against the philistinism of the colleges. In our experiences (E.A.L. and N.S.) in directing a parent group, it is notable how difficult it was initially to get the parents to stop blaming someone else or to stop talking in a condescending, knowledgeable way about their childrens' difficulties. As they explore more their own personality problems, we are struck by their difficulty (under the facile "what have we done wrong?") in accepting responsibility. To them it is always really someone else's fault. The trouble their children are having in the world and with their parents seems an extension of the same difficulty the parents had in their world and with their parents.

We have been discussing these students and their families using a variety of psychiatric metaphors; character structure, psychodynamics, family homeostasis, family ethology. A brief clinical example may illustrate these different dimensions. They are not "levels." There is no pejorative implication of shallowness or depth. They are only different metaphors facilitating our understanding of a continuum of experience.

> A boy we shall call Ronald drops out of his third year of college, still maintaining good marks. He returns home and takes up the dropout stance. He finds himself caught again in the usual exchange with his father, which has gone on as long as anyone can remember, to wit, his father encourages him to take up any variety of activities, Ronald responds apathetically. His father cajoles, bribes, buys expensive equipment, hires instructors, and so forth. Ronald starts the activity. Father participates helpfully. Ronald flies into a rage and quits. The father gets him boxing lessons, tennis lessons, music lessons. Ronald is unable to do anything without the father's urging but soon quits because he's being "pushed." After many months of sitting about the house, Ronald decides (on his own) to take driving lessons. He enrolls at a school and takes several lessons. The father is delighted. To "encourage him," the father takes him out one afternoon in his car for a supplementary lesson. We have the usual denouement. Ronald flies into a rage at his father, almost smashes the car and quits lessons-with the father in despair.

Let us examine these data from the point of view of the metaphors we have suggested.

1. *Characterological*: We have a severe passive-aggressive personality disorder. The boy demands help, responding hostilely to it when it is offered. At the first frustration he reacts with impotence and rage, directed against the poor helper, who fails to meet his standards for magical competence.

2. *Dyadic*: He and the father have an intense sadomasochistic exchange. His father has directed, interfered with, and dominated every move the boy has made. Under his mask of benevolent concern, he cannot bear it that his son do something on his own. He interferes and directs until the boy flies into a rage and attacks him. Then he assumes an obsequious masochistic posture. For example, he is so involved with the boy that he checks the garbage can to see how much of his dinner he has eaten. Although the father had ample

experience to indicate that if he became involved in the driving lessons there would be a disaster, he could not resist the temptation Nor could the boy resist accepting his involvement, milking the father for his own needs to avoid commitment and responsibility and using the father as excuse to exercise his sadistic power.

3. On an intricate *homeostatic* level this repeated exchange between father and son serves to maintain the family integrity. It diverts attention from and provides a vicarious substitute for the severe lack of mothering provided by the wife. Both father and son get some gratification from each other, distract attention from the mother's affective silence, and make it possible for the father to maintain the illusion that he is satisfied and has a good marriage. The father dissociates his own immense dependency yearnings by playing the role of the helper. If son or wife step out of their complementary roles, he gets panicky, precipitates a crisis, and forces them back into line. It is interesting, too, that if the boy begins to get reasonable, the father's dependency breaks through. He begins to depend on the boy, using him as a confidant, appealing to him for sustenance. The son becomes frightened, in his turn provokes a fight and they both avoid awareness of dependency needs. To elaborate on the driving incident which precipitated the crisis: the father took the boy out, after some urging, at dusk, in his large luxury limousine, and over the boy's protests suggested he drive on a two-way brightly lighted main thoroughfare; having the experience of only a few lessons, blinded by oncoming headlights, the boy panicked.

4. From the point of view of *family style*, we know from a three generation examination of the family that the father had little direct experience of an appropriate fathering role. His own father was an austere and distant man. He himself, outside of business performance, is rather inept socially. In this family, as a subculture, one might say that there is a stylistic failure to implement appropriate learning procedures. The father cannot teach his son how to function in the outside world. All he can do is "show confidence in him"-that is, whatever the situation, no matter how inappropriate to the boy's real skills or level of accomplishment, the father encourages him to go on. Of course, the boy falls on his face and then turns in rage on the father, whom he sees as unreliable. This kind of distrust of the helper is something the therapist working with dropouts comes to experience and it is not entirely a distortion. The patient has had much experience with gratuitous encouragement without real help. One might say the father took him driving to "show his confidence" under conditions well beyond the boy's skill. The family ethos prescribes that confidence, admiration, and faith in

the child will make him successful. Criticism is not allowed. In the family, with the father's short stopping, the boy can function adequately. In the outside world, of course, this breaks down.

None of this emphasis on family dynamics and ethos is intended to minimize the importance of the intrapsychic life, particularly of the fantasy life of the patient. Nor are we proselytizing conjoint family therapy or group therapy. However, that therapist who thinks in terms of the family in addition to the intrapsychic life of the patient will be inclined to hear things slightly differently. For example, the same boy we have discussed has sexual fantasies in which he is tied to a bedstead, whipped and sexually stimulated by a scantily-clad girl. He is ashamed and disgusted by these fantasies. To be sure, they are masochistic and guilt-ridden. They are also in defense against his markedly hostile feelings toward women. But they are also utterly consistent with an important aspect of the *family system*. To wit, one must deny any interest or self-seeking for pleasure. The other person must be provoked into forcing something you really want on you, *against your will*. This is the way to get taken care of without being overwhelmed or overprotected. Also, it renders irrelevant one's incompetence in the techniques of pursuing girls.

These different formulations of this clinical example (and there are certainly many more) emphasize the multidimensionality of the problem and at the same time the one striking common denominator, that is, the unreliability of the manifest message, "Father wants to help". This is, we strongly suspect, the reason for our getting caught, in our work, in our countertransference sense of dishonesty. The patient has learned to distrust both his own authenticity and that of the other person. He suspects, with good reason, that he fulfills intense, disguised emotional needs for other members of the family.

In the well integrated families described by Murphey and Silber children are valued by the parents, but are not essential to their psychic well-being.[23] The family can let the student go and moreover is competent to supply him with the instrumental techniques for survival in the outside world. In the family of the schizophrenic, the pressures on the child to participate in a tenuous homeostatic balance are so frighteningly immense and basically irrational that emotional disturbance appears within the family group and may in deed be vital to the maintenance of the sanity of the other family members.[9,26] That is, in the schizophrenic family, the pseudo-mutuality is maintained by reifying the child's role as the "sick one" or "crazy one." In the neurotic family, the child plays the role of the "bad one" or the "unappreciative one," forcing him to internalize his guilt. In these families, the pseudo-mutuality is maintained by insisting they are all content and well. When this breaks down in contact with the outside world, they tend to see their child, the dropout, as the "unpredictable one."

We might ask why is the college epoch so crucial? Why do difficulties not appear earlier? There is usually a history of some prior school troubles and/or peer difficulties, but college is actually the first time it is permissible to fail outright. If dropping out is a choice, it cannot be exercised until a viable occasion arrives. Kubie quoted St. Augustine rather neatly when he said that the innocence of children depends more on the shortness of their limbs than the purity of their hearts.[15] The dropout drops out when he can!

What, finally, are the implications of all this for psychoanalytic therapy? These families are characterized by unauthenticity, pseudo- mutuality, discontent, and masked rebelliousness. Moreover, the members are components of very powerful, self-perpetuating homeostatic systems in which symptomatic distress is directed outside the family, to wit, "Go outside if you're going to be sick." These are, we think, the preconditions for the sociopathic solution. The therapist will find himself sucked into this vortex, incorporated into a system where verbal communication is unreliable, help is ambivalent and often inappropriate, and appearance of congeniality must be maintained. Ergo, he is enjoined not to establish a pseudo-mutuality with the patient based on his own need to be healthy, happy, or right. Aligning oneself with the patient against his family can become an inadvertent consequence of exploring the family dynamics, a form of pseudo-mutuality which says to the patient, "Let's you and I get along well together. It is the others who make trouble." He must respect the patient's distrust of offered help, which has often been an invitation to jump off the barn roof carrying an umbrella, and he must not be dismayed by the intense tribal loyalties which make the patient opaque to insight.

The primary strategy of therapy is this: It does not much matter what the therapist says, what metaphor or theoretical system he employs; what does matter is his transferential posture, that is, the extent to which he and the patient can avoid recapitulating the family stance. For example, an interpretation which focuses on a characterological pattern of the student, namely, how his grandiosity affects his writing a term paper may be immensely effective. Not so much because of the accuracy of the content, but because the patient's family always treated school difficulties by saying, "You're very smart and we believe in you." Just such a directed criticism may be new to him. Yet, the same statement to a student with the same difficulty will be less than worthless if his family experience has been of much intellectual analysis and criticism, but of neither trust nor sufficient confidence to permit him to go off on his own. The patient believes not the words, but the transaction; not the content but the intent. The therapist often will find himself incorporated in a transference which is a recapitulation of the family situation. He will, willy-nilly, experience the role of the parent with all its concomitant exasperation and impotence. It is vital therefore, that he be able to open the system to new data, to deal with the patient in a different, more potent way. Above all, he must, throughout the course of this largely nonverbal exchange, provide a verbal commentary, much like the subtitles that flash across the bottom of a foreign movie, teaching the patient to trust and use a mutually validated language.

Therapy then, proceeds as a ballet of changing nonverbal patterns. One might call this an *action* transference; it is not acting out in the transference, which is another thing entirely. Acting out is behavior which is intended to belie or obfuscate a verbal transaction in the therapy. It is in the service of resistance. These patients communicate by action because words are unreliable in their experience. Language has been, for them, more a ritual for the maintenance of tribal intactness than a means of communication.

To conclude: We have attempted to view dropping out as a manifestation of a larger social ill, coming increasingly to the notice of psychotherapists. The antecedents for this "sociopathic" action can be found in a particular family structure, which we have delineated in some detail. Much of what we have presented is, of course, not completely documented yet and requires further validation through on-campus studies and certainly more extensive family studies. Consideration of the family as a psychosocial unit with its own imperatives, and the patient as a participating member of that group regardless of physical propinquity, throws much light on the specificity of symptom choice and on the often paradoxical relationship between successful social performance and degree of psychiatric disturbance.

REFERENCES

1. Ackerman, N. W., *The Psychodynamics of Family Life* (New York: Basic Books, 1958).
2. -, in a discussion of "Identity and Ego Autonomy in Adolescence" by R. Shapiro, in *Science and Psychoanalysis*, ed. J. Masserman (New York: Grune & Stratton, 1966), p. 25.
3. -, "Family Psychotherapy-Theory and Practice," *Amer. J. Psychother.*, 20

(1966), 405.

4. Akeret, R., and Stockhamer, N., "Countertransference Reactions to College Drop-Outs", *Amer.J. Psychother.*, 20 (1965), 622.

5. Bieber, I., *Homosexuality*, (New York: Basic Books, 1962).

6. Erikson, E. H., "Youth: Fidelity and Diversity," *Daedalus: J. Amer. Acad. Arts & Sci.* (Winter 1962), 5.

7. -"The Problem of Ego Identity", *J. Amer. Psychoanal. Ass.*, 4 (1956) 56.

8. Farnsworth, D. S., "We're Wasting Brain Power," *J. Nat. Educ. Ass.*, (March 1959).

9. Feiner, A., and Levenson, E., "Sacrifice: One Aspect in the Meaningfulness of the Act of Dropping Out,' College Dropout Project of the William Alanson White Institute, unpublished manuscript.

10. Ford, D., and Urban, H., "College Dropouts: Successes or Failures?" in *The College Dropout and the Utilization of Talent*, eds. L. Pervin, L. Reik, and W. Dalrymple, (Princeton, N.J.: Princeton University Press, 1966), pp. 83-100.

11. Keniston, K., *The Uncommitted*, (New York: Harcourt, Brace & World,1960).

12. -, "College Students and Children in Developmental Institutions." *Children*, 14, (1967), 4.

13. Kohn, M., and Levenson, E., "Some Characteristics of a Group of Bright, Emotionally Disturbed College Dropouts," *J. Amer. Coll. Health Ass.*, 14 (1965), 78.2.

-, "Differences Between Accepted and Rejected Patients in a Treatment Project of College Dropouts," *J. Psychol.*, 63 (1966), 143.

15. Kubie L., "The Ontogeny of The Dropout Problem," in *The College Drop Out and The Utilization of Talent*, eds. L. Pervin, L. Reik, and W. Dalrymple, (Princeton. N.J.: Princeton Univ. Press, 1966), pp. 23-35.

16. Levenson, E., "College Dropout: A Manifestation of Family Homeostasis," presented at a meeting of the *American Orthopsychiatric Association*, March 1964.

17. -, "A Treatment Facility for College Dropouts," *Ment. Hyg.*, 49 (1965), 413.

18. -, "Why Do They Drop Out?" *Teaching & Learning* (1965), 1.

19. -, "Some Socio-Cultural Issues in the Etiology and Treatment of College Dropouts," in *The College Dropout and the Utilization of Talent*, eds. L.Pervin, L. Reik, and W. Dalrymple, (Princeton, N.J.: Princeton University Press, 1966), pp. 189-206.

20. Levenson, E., and Kohn, M., "A Demonstration Clinic for College

Dropouts," *College Health*, 12 (1964), 382.

21. Levenson, J. S., "Observations of Similar Attitudes Among the Families of College Dropouts, College Dropout Project of the William Alan White Institute, unpublished manuscript.

22. Lidz, T., Fleck, S., and Cornielson, A., *Schizophrenia and the Family*. (New York, Int. Univ. Press, 1965).

23. Murphey, E., Silber E., et al. "Development of Autonomy and Parent-Child Interaction in Late Adolescence," *Dept. of Health, Education Welfare, U.S. Public Health Service*, Bethesda, Md., (mimeographed).

24. Pervin, L., "The Later Academic, Vocational and Personal Success of College Dropouts," in *The College Drop-Out and the Utilization of Talent*. (Princeton, N.J.: Princeton Univ. Press, 1966), pp. 37-62.

25. Pervin, L., Reik, L., and Dalrymple. W., *The College Drop-Out and the Utilization of Talent*. (Princeton, N.J.: Princeton Univ. Press, 1966)

26. Searles, H. F., *Collected Papers on Schizophrenia and Related Subjects*; (New York: Int. Univ. Press, 1965).

27. Singer, E., "Identity vs Identification, a Thorny Psychological Issue," *Rev. Existent. Psychol. Psychiat., 5 (1965), 160.*

CHAPTER FIFTEEN
THE PARANOID-SCHIZOID
POSITION
IN EARLY ADOLESCENCE

Owen Lewis

The divergence of clinical psychoanalytic theory and metapsychology has been described by many authors and perhaps most elaborately by George Klein (1976). This divergence is probably most extreme during the stage of development of early adolescence. Although there are a number of well-articulated psychoanalytic theories of adolescent development (Blos, 1962a; Jacobson, 1964; Erikson, 1968), there is certainly not a coherent clinical theory of psychoanalytic treatments at this stage. At best, technique is described in terms of modifications of the adult model of psychoanalysis.

In this paper I will be suggesting a model of analytic treatment of the early adolescent drawn from a formulation of development based on object relations theory. I will begin by describing the clinical presentation of two early adolescents who showed marked pathological regressions. A formulation of their pathology will be presented based on Melanie Klein's concept of the paranoid-schizoid position. The implications of this formulation of these adolescents' treatments will be discussed. Finally, I will suggest ways in which this approach applies more generally to psychoanalytic treatment of the early adolescent.

The concept of a normative regression in early adolescence has been described from multiple vantage points: ego structure, drives, a second separation-individuation phase, a reworking of the oedipal complex, and object relations. (Katan, 1951; A. Freud, 1958; Blos, 1962a; Jacobson, 1964). Where the normal adolescent during the early phases of adolescence will show and continuous fluctuation in the degree and quality of regression, gratification, defense, and adaptation, there are those adolescents who find themselves in the grips of a regression beyond which they cannot develop. In the broadest sense, this is what is meant by a developmental breakdown. Whatever pathogenic stresses the adolescent may be facing, the stress of his or her own development is predominant.

Laufer and Laufer (1984, p. 23) have described a number of ways in which such breakdowns may manifest themselves symptomatically. These include withdrawal from peers, compulsive masturbation with perverse actions, attacks on parents, a new onset of school phobia, denial of the physical changes of puberty with an attempt to change the body, and self-harming or suicidal gestures. Where behaviors are overt and rebellious, as in the pseudoindependent disregard of restrictions which is so common, or in the pseudo heterosexual behaviors of early adolescence (Blos, 1962a), the defensive functioning against the regressive instinct can be gleaned. In those adolescents, however, who manifest internalizing symptoms with overt behaviors of withdrawal and avoidance, the nature of their regressions may be less apparent and more entrenched than is initially apparent. The cases of two adolescents whom I will be presenting typify this class of problem.

Lisa was 15 when she was coerced into a psychiatric consultation. Towards the end of the ninth grade she had begun missing school and over the summer began to experience difficulty traveling without accompaniment. When I first saw her in the late fall, she had been unable to attend school entirely for several months.

She made it clear from the first consultation that she was uninterested in treatment. She was not disturbed by the school problem, mildly disturbed by the traveling problem, but most of all bothered by the shape of her nose. She was unable to look at her face's full reflection but with a small compact mirror would study her nose from every angle. During the summer she had been told that she was an Edie Sedgewick look-alike, Edie Sedgewick being a deceased model and avant-garde actress made famous by Andy Warhol. Her nose was the one feature which she feared distinguished her from Edie. Over that summer she had begun collecting information on Edie and read the recently published biography like a Bible. In fact, Lisa was often able to travel alone when she carried the biography or her scrapbook of Edie articles.

What was striking was her ability to recount to me almost every detail of Edie's life and almost nothing of her own. "Typical psychiatry questions" at best bored her. More often, she was at a complete loss of words in response to any question that touched on her thoughts or feelings about her phobias, body distortions, or relationships to family or friends. In fact Lisa decided to pursue treatment with me because I offered to purchase a copy of the biography "for the office." The importance of this decision was highlighted by an incident during the second year of treatment. Lisa's agoraphobia and school phobia were generally improved but transiently recurring. Halfway to my office, traveling on her own, Lisa panicked. Rather than turn back, she was able to continue on knowing that a copy of the biography awaited her. This she borrowed in order to return home.

I came to appreciate her inability to talk about her problematic thoughts and feelings as a symptom in itself. Although the external phobic symptoms were clear, the same process was at work in relation to her own thoughts and feelings. An incident 6 months into treatment demonstrated this. Entering the session, Lisa confessed that she had stopped up the toilet in the waiting room lavatory. While waiting, she had tried on her glasses for the first time m many months, was horrified by her complete facial reflection, broke her glasses into bits and flushed them away. This was the first I learned that Lisa even wore glasses. Although it was becoming safer for her to see, she had unfocused the world by her self-imposed myopia. Denial of this extreme has its counterpart in a psychic denial, hence her absolute inability to discuss thoughts and feelings in the usual way.

Kevin at 13 presented in a manner similar to Lisa. He had skirmishes with transient school phobia since the age of 9 with intermittent psychiatric treatment that proved frustrating both to him and the previous psychiatrist who "couldn't get him to talk about his feelings." A new and overzealous school psychologist made some determined home visits, with the result that Kevin stopped attending school altogether. When he first saw me in consultation he had been home for some 8 months. His inarticulateness about the symptom was more severe even than Lisa's. When pushed to express himself, he became nearly apoplectically red in the face. Like Lisa, he too entered the first consultation with a book in hand. His interest was in comic books, superheroes, and horror movies. As mute as he was about his fears, he could talk at length about the super heroes. He knew, actually, nearly every fact about every superhero in just about every described galaxy in the Marvel Comics universe. The superheroes and the latest horror movies served as the basis for our conversations.

Kevin, too, showed his version of Lisa's self-imposed myopia. Some 2 years into treatment, when Kevin was beginning to express an interest in girls, he reported that while walking down the street a good-looking girl had smiled at him and he went back into tunnel-vision. He was most surprised that I didn't know what he meant. On questioning, I learned that for at least the first year of treatment he was able to travel around only when he used tunnel vision, by which he meant focusing only on a thin straight line ahead of him and tuning all else out. At this point, tunnel vision was no longer generally needed. He also revealed that he had also navigated about with a system of mental maps that delineated safe and unsafe areas. In retrospect he was functioning in a state of generalized agoraphobia, as well as the school phobia, but his adaptation to the former had quickly become ego syntonic.

Treatment with Lisa and Kevin quickly fell into a routine. With

Lisa, for many months we read together, each from his copy of the Edie Sedgewick biography. She'd tell me to look at page so and so, where we'd discuss an aspect of her life, or discuss how she appeared in a given photograph. As time went on, we shifted to a discussion of Lisa's looks, often discussing her appearance in photos of herself that she brought in. Although she did not give up her distortions of her own physical appearance for the longest time, the distortions lessened in reality to her. With Kevin, I began by asking him endless questions about the superheroes. This evolved into my giving him "superhero quizzes" on which he always got an "A+" and which soon had an effect on his fear of test-taking in school. When I had exhausted my repertoire of superhero questions, I suggested that he bring in comics that he owned doubles of, and we did oral readings together, dividing up the parts. Sessions might also begin with his straight-faced recitation of the gory details of the most recent horror movie.

Although the treatments went on for several years, both adolescents were back in school within 4 months after treatment started. Consolidation of this gain, of course, required a much longer period of time. An explanation of these gains lies both in the conceptualization of the pathology and of the treatment.

With no more history than what has been given, and it is obvious how difficult obtaining a personal history from these adolescents would be at this stage, one already has a great deal of information. The subsequent clinical procedure will necessarily derive from the conception of analysis at this stage. If the model is essentially that of adult analysis with modification, one will proceed cautiously to identify conflictual themes in the material. For instance, there are aspects of the relationship to the hero which represent the ego-ideal, yet the relationship is dependent and the admired traits are passively acquired. With Edie, these traits involved grandiosely, if not magically, acquired fame and admiration. With the superheroes, these traits involved strength and overcoming threats of destruction. Another example of such a conflict is that of sexual identity. These figures allowed for a postponement of choice for the adolescent. Edie, although female, is thin, boyish, and androgynous. Among the female superheroes are many muscle-bound and angular women whose strength matches any man's. These conflicts clearly cannot be addressed as one would an adult with well-developed ego and cognitive capacities.

Defense analysis is a cornerstone of the classical approach. Here we see, first and foremost, denial in the visual symptoms. Denial is, of course, one of the earliest and most pathological of defenses. We also see projection, which is inherent in the phobic symptom. Along with this, there is a primitive splitting, seen in the elaboration of safe and unsafe areas, blatantly good and bad characters, and thinking that in general is dominated by these binary functions. Projective identification is also operative, most obviously in the attribute of the hero. Drawing the adolescent's attention to the pathology of his defenses is, however, impossible. We are not addressing an individual with generally more evolved defenses who has pockets of maladaptive pathological defenses. These defenses are dominating most of the adolescents' operations.

If, for the most part, the content of the conflict or the types of defense against it have been excluded from the analyst's comments in the clinical encounter, what then guides the clinical encounter? It is, I believe, the quality of the therapeutic relationship as it evolves, and the underlying, developmentally determined, capacity for relationship.

At the start of treatment, Lisa's and Kevin's primary and most involved relationship was with the hero. In the early years of treatment, Lisa usually had one best friend who was just like her by her own description, but who quickly fell out of favor. Kevin, at this point, had withdrawn from peer relationships except for visits arranged by his mother. Their day-in and day-out concerns with the hero. In the therapeutic relationship, I was allowed at first to observe this, approve of it, and share in it as time went on but not allowed to be curious about their feelings, thoughts, or wishes outside of their interest in the hero. They were each extremely reliable about coming to sessions. There was never any question about the importance of the treatment to them, but neither was there any expression of its importance.

The nature of this relationship can be understood as schizoid. that is, one in which there is an extreme of dependency as well as a denial of dependency. Because the dependency was experienced in relation to a fictive character, there was protection against the self-dissolution experienced in merging with another. This is akin to the phenomenon Anna Freud (1958) described as a state of primary identification in which the relief of the regression can be only short-lived because of the deeper anxiety of emotional surrender. Fairbairn (1940) described three features of schizoid phenomena: an attitude of omnipotence, an attitude of isolation and detachment, and a preoccupation with inner reality. The omnipotence is evident in the extreme control exerted both in the therapeutic relationship and in relationship to the hero. The detachment and isolation permeated actual relationships. The extent of the visual symptoms is indicative of the degree to which external reality was excluded. From Fairbairn, too, we learn that when there is an overinvest in internal reality, the act of giving leads to inner impoverishment, and hence there is a predominance of taking in relation to others. The inability of these adolescents to respond to the analyst's questions may be understood in this context. What they each wanted first was external approval and support of their inner fantasies. On one occasion when Lisa hazarded a dream, my attempts to pursue an interpretation were met with a rebuke: Couldn't I just appreciate her dream?

Melanie Klein (1946) expanded on the operations and etiology of schizoid states in her concept of the paranoid-schizoid position. This concept describes more broadly the psychology of the first object relationship. As originally delineated (see also Segal, 1981), this corresponded to the first 6 months of life. Developmentally, this relational position was followed by the depressive position (Klein, 1935). Before I elaborate on these concepts as they relate to adolescent regressions, I wish to cite Ogden's reference to these positions as "distinctive states of being" that "constitute enduring, fundamental components of all subsequent psychological states" (1986, p. 5). More broadly, he sees the paranoid-schizoid position as representing the transition "from the purely biological to psychological experience" and the depressive position as representing the transition "from the impersonal psychological to subjective experience." Understood in this way, regression to one of these positions will be taken to mean a regression to a more fundamental and primitive way of organizing experience and relationships not literally a regression to the experience of a 6 month old.

A Kleinian position may be specified in terms of (1) the nature of the object relationship, (2) the nature of the defenses, (3) the nature of the dominant anxiety, and, related to this, (4) the attendant set of fantasies. In the paranoid-schizoid position, the object relationship is in essence schizoid as described by Fairbairn The defenses, as previously described, are those considered the most primitive. A particular emphasis in the Kleinian concept of a relational position is the nature of the anxiety.

Paranoid, or persecutory anxiety, refers to the anxiety of destruction or annihilation. It is felt more powerfully as an overwhelmingly dreadful force and is qualitatively distinct from other anxieties. For Klein, it exists in conjunction with the operation of a set of fantasies involving the wish to destroy the frustrating object, the projection of retaliation, and the weakening inherent in complete surrender to the satisfying object. Whether this set of fantasies is repressed, as with Lisa, or displaced, as with Kevin, any discussion of the fantasies in direct relation to the adolescent is to reify them. Their subjective experience, however, can be seen to be dominated by this overwhelming emotion. They were hounded at every turn by their fears. An appreciation of this quality of anxiety must inform every intervention. For Freud the situations which give rise to anxiety were specified, and the quantity of anxiety was specified, but there was little attention to the quality of anxiety. The full extent of the generalized phobic withdrawals shown by Lisa and Kevin could not be appreciated for some time because they refrained or were unable to discuss their symptoms and because they rapidly incorporated many of their symptoms in an ego-syntonic manner. Some prior conception, therefore, is needed which elucidates the quality and extent of the anxiety by which one can surmise the subjective experience which is essentially unspeakable. The descriptions of persecutory anxiety provide this.

The concept of the paranoid-schizoid position offers a unified approach to the phenomena. From pathological defenses, one may assume the presence of persecutory anxiety and schizoid relatedness. From more evident schizoid detachment, one may similarly assume the presence of the other elements. When one then considers the nature of treatment that will unfold, the concept of a relational position will attune the analyst to how it is possible to relate to the individual. An individual is in the given "position." He must be encountered in this "position." One must speak the language of the "position." The analyst's automatic questions- How do you feel? What were you thinking when . . . ?-translate without empathic connotation but with intrusion, threat, and violence. The adolescent who cannot use a real mirror is in no position to use the "therapeutic mirror."

As can be seen, my use of object relations theory to illuminate these early adolescent regressions concerns the structure, not the content, of the relational regression. Almost all theories of adolescent development describe a shift in object relations. The decathexis of the primary object relationships in order to make nonincestuous libidinal attachments in adolescence was first described by Freud (1905) in "Three Essays on Sexuality." Katan (1951) made this shift explicit in a process she termed object removal. Other writers (A. Freud, 1958; Blos, 1962a; Jacobson 1964) have contributed to an understanding of this process. A formulation of these regressions in terms of the paranoid-schizoid position, however, emphasizes the nature of the relationship that is possible at this stage. Since all psychoanalysis proceeds through, the therapeutic relationship, it can be seen that the structure of the relational regression must guide treatment.

Returning to the treatments of Lisa and Kevin, the program of the sessions changed little for over a year. Although the joint readings gave way to broader discussions of their heroes, these were never self-reflective in any way. As can be seen the adolescents exerted extensive control over the sessions. This might be said to mirror the more primitive grandiosity of control of the primary object, but since the adolescents had virtually withdrawn from the world of relationships, it was a necessary precondition for a reentry into actual and viable relationships. The control exerted in the relationship to the fictive hero was gradually extended to the figure of the analyst. The act of joint reading allowed for an extensive, but symbolic, regression reminiscent of bedtime story reading. This was followed with the more active reading by the adolescent. The entire process, however, remained under the control of the adolescent who had, of course, chosen the story.

The formulation of the paranoid-schizoid position informs us too that the nature of the phobia is not what might first assume to be reflecting separation anxiety as many writers have described in, relation to school phobia (Johnson et al., 1941; Coolidge et al., 1957; Eisenberg, 1958; Sperling, 1967). Separation anxiety assumes a relatively complete internal object representation and would be understood in Kleinian terms as pathology related to the depressive position. With these adolescents, the fear was not one of being away from someone, but rather one of being out in the world. In this sense, the hero can be understood to be what might be termed an identity symbol. Thus, there is not only the relationship to the hero, but the adolescent is the hero who is successfully out in the world. In his story, 'the adolescent sees his own personal conflicts impersonally. Yet it can also be said that the adolescent creates the identity symbol. To disregard the identity symbol is to disregard the adolescent. It is the only way he can speak about himself and his wish to be back in the world. Attention then to the identity symbol serves to usher the adolescent back into a relationship and back into the world. In his extended, regressed control of the analyst, the adolescent transfers his "primary identification" with the hero to the analyst and thereby defuses it. In terms of aggressive drives, the rebuffed personal question the imperfect analyst must now and then hazards experienced as a violating intrusion. But it also serves to subtly challenge the split between the ideal and the persecuting, and this leads to a differentiation between interpersonal assertiveness and the more virulent forms of feared aggression.

For the analyst, engagement in a relationship that is predominantly schizoid is intermittently, but necessarily, boring. His curiosity must be curtailed and his sense of improvisation guarded. The boredom is an essential aspect of the experience and must be welcomed. In time, the adolescent's own experience of boredom will allow him to begin to challenge his own phobically circumscribed limitations.

Having admonished a requisite curtailment of one's usual analytic curiosity, I have thus postponed presenting any description of the developmental hazards experienced by Lisa and Kevin which probably gave rise to the massive regressions in early adolescence. Between the ages of 3 and 4, Lisa's parents separated. Although they had been rather dedicated parents previously and were so subsequently, for this period of time Lisa was virtually abandoned by them and left with a series of friends and caretakers. Although there were no reported regressions in language or self-care behaviors, descriptions of her at the time suggest a depression. Around the age of 7 she experienced mild separation anxiety and recurrent nightmares. For Kevin, the nature of his relationship with his father posed a developmental hazard. His father was an unusually unemotional and distant figure whose main interaction with his son at home was to criticize anything that disrupted his routine or interfered with the orderliness he required. Their one "fun" activity, from a very early age on, was to go shooting together.

There is, of course, much more to say about each of their developmental histories, but I give this information to show how irrelevant these facts are to the clinical process. Lisa's terrifying separations in the past were of course inherent in the present fears. Similarly with Kevin, the overstimulation of aggression with his father in the past was inherent in the present clashing of the superheroes or in the compulsive watching of horror movies. The fears are so overwhelming, however, that no extraneous elements can be introduced. The defenses are operative to contain the emergency in the present. The phobic symptoms which separate the safe from the unsafe for the adolescent carve out for him a livable niche.

Transference does not exist discretely. To describe the transferences as part-object transferences is of course correct, but this suggests that the parts of the object in the transference may be delineated. Splitting describes the defensive operation which, like the overt phobic symptom, attempts to separate safe from unsafe, good from bad. However, the unsafe and the bad cannot be tangled with. They are cast out. Repression has usually failed, to be supplanted by denial. These adolescents do not challenge or criticize the analyst. Instead, they fix him in a position that is rather distantly aligned with the good and safe projections. In this position he is kept from eliciting the terrifying anxiety that is almost always rampant. His goodness and safeness is of an impersonal nature, that is, it exists via the goodness he has allowed to be ascribed to him.

The splitting that is usually described in the borderline patient is different from this process. Borderline splitting is probably closer to vacillations of idealization and denigrations which assume a more coherent self which can feel disappointment and a more coherent view of the object as one capable of carrying out an idealized function. When denigration and disappointment become manifest in the clinical interaction, a more advanced stage of object relations has been reached. In Kleinian terminology, these experiences are part of the depressive position. At this point, the analyst approaches being viewed as a more complete object, however distorted, and he may now attempt to interpretatively describe the distortions, the clinical interactions, and affects or ideas out of the patient's immediate consciousness. At this point, too, seemingly paradoxically, the adolescent becomes not so good a patient, more frequently missing sessions, coming late, wanting to change times.

Because interpretation assumes a higher level of self and object integration, as well as more involved cognitive and emotional functioning, interpretation is not a useful therapeutic mode for the patient predominantly in the paranoid-schizoid position. In fact, the analyst oriented solely toward interpretation may impede the adolescent's recovery. Rather the emphasis must remain on the adolescent's experience in a relationship in which he is given extreme control and whose forays into a relationship are met with cautious appreciation. A formulation of the type of regression manifested by Lisa and Kevin in terms of the paranoid-schizoid position emphasizes the nature of the anxiety, the primitive defensive operations, and the quality of object relations. It should be pointed out, however, that the therapeutic approach I have suggested is at variance with Klein's (1932) recommendations regarding adolescent analysis. She allowed for few technical modifications at this stage.

In summary then, this approach to the analytic treatment of the severely regressed adolescent suggests treating the adolescent, at least initially, as one would a schizoid character. Features of this approach include (1) the importance of the adolescent's control of the therapeutic relationship; (2) the fragility of relationships and the degree of withdrawal from relationships; (3) the adolescent's creation of an identity symbol which represents some aspect of the idealized self functioning in the world, the adolescent's attempt to reengage in real relationships, and comprises as well his regressed relationship to a primary object; (4) the requisite curtailment of the analyst's curiosity with the attendant countertransference response of boredom; and (5) the relative contraindication of an interpretative approach until evidence of phenomena of the depressive position are manifest. Above all, it is important to conceptualize the clinical process as derived from, and specific for. this set of psychological operations. not as deviations from an analytic process specific for more mature psychological operations or as preparation for future analytic work which, l believe, guarantees a poor attunement between analyst and adolescent.

Thus far, I have been discussing a formulation and treatment pertaining to two adolescents who manifested extreme developmental, although not psychotic, regressions. I would like to raise the question whether this particular formulation of their regression has relevance to the normative regression of this developmental stage, and if, correspondingly, this model of treatment is applicable more generally to other disorders arising at this stage.

The concept of a normative regression in early adolescence is well established (A. Freud, 1958; Blos, 1962a; Jacobson, 1964). This regression has been described in terms of an increase in pregenital drives and in terms of the relative weakness of the ego in relation to the emerging drives. This necessarily involves a regression to more primitive mechanisms of defense which has been noted as an essential aspect of the paranoid-schizoid position.

The second important aspect of the paranoid-schizoid position entails the nature of the object relations described as schizoid. Is there evidence for this in the normally developing adolescent? The importance of the group to the early adolescent is manifestly evident (Group for the Advancement of Psychiatry, 1968). Among the reasons for this have been included the need to replace the family allegiance. Group identification also involves relatively impersonal and less intimate relationships. Individual choice, decision making, and preference are suspended and supplanted by a conformity that allows for any individual to substitute for another. This can be seen as reflecting a basically schizoid manner of relating. As one 14-year-old boy with a mild conduct disturbance put it when I asked him if he ever remembered his dreams: "I don't tell my dreams to anybody. In fact, you'll never catch me telling anything personal to anybody."

Although she does not use the term schizoid to describe the early adolescent's object relations, Geleerd (1961) has detailed the normative process in adolescence as a partial regressive to the undifferentiated phase of object relations. This concept is developed in terms of degree of dependence on the love objects and the fusion of inner and outer experience and can be seen to be directly related to the concept of the paranoid-schizoid position.

Finally there is the particular nature of the anxiety manifest in this position which has been described as persecutory. Clearly, most adolescents do not manifest the quantity nor quality of the anxiety experienced by Lisa and Kevin. An emotion, however that is universal at this stage is self-consciousness. Is there an adolescent who at some point has not cringed at his own reflection or felt the eyes of the whole class sneering at him as he entered late? Self-consciousness is, I believe, the normal manifestation of persecutory anxiety. The experience of a normative and usually transient regression to the paranoid-schizoid position is also captured in Blos's discussion of adolescent acting out: "The outside world appears to the adolescent, at least in certain aspects, as the mirror image of his internal reality, with its conflicts threats, and comforts; his inner world is thus summarily experienced as external. Every adolescent is brushed-even if for brief moments-by paranoid ideation" (1962a, p. 268). This is, in essence, a phobic process which can only occur with extensive projection and omnipotent denial.

Other writers have reflected their recognition of this process. Katan (1951) described the process of object removal in adolescents whereby an individual irreversibly breaks the primary object ties to the parents in order to make nonincestuous attachments. What is often overlooked in this much quoted paper is that in her description of the process of object removal she compares a 14 year-old girl's flight from treatment during her first love relationship (when the process of object removal was being realized) with a 41-year-old woman's agoraphobia which had been present since the age of 14. Although object removal is the normative process and agoraphobia the pathologic, both entail a phobic process and at least transient schizoid object relations. For Katan, this phobic process is ubiquitous. In the same essay (p. 50) she writes: "Slight agoraphobia as an acute symptom seems to constitute a normal transitory stage in young girls." It is in such observations that one can detect a normative return to the paranoid-schizoid position. Although Katan does not comment on the nature of the object relations accompanying this phobic process, Segal (1954) has expanded on schizoid mechanisms underlying phobia formation.

Returning to Fairbairn, who pioneered the exploration of the psychology of schizoid phenomena, we find a reference to the relevance of schizoid operations to adolescent psychopathology. He described several categories where overt schizoid conditions may be found. Among these is "the schizoid state, or transient schizoid episode-a category under which, in my opinion, a considerable proportion of adolescent 'nervous breakdowns' fall" (1940, p.

4).

Thus there are many indications that the concept of the paranoid-schizoid position is more generally applicable to the normative experience of the early adolescent. Reviewing in this light some of the discussion of analytic technique in early adolescence, the disparate recommendations of various writers can be seen to reflect a more unified approach.

Geleerd states: "The ego of the [early] adolescent is already so threatened by the increased id drives that a very little over eagerness on the analyst's part may be too overwhelming" (1957, p. 273). This corresponds to what I have described as the requisite curtailment of curiosity on the part of the analyst.

Laufer and Laufer (1984) have cautioned against interpreting the preadolescent past until the adolescent breakdown, in its own terms, has been understood. An understanding of the present must be constructed before any reconstruction of early childhood is possible. To judge from their numerous examples, this inevitably waits until, at the earliest, the late adolescent years. This corresponds, as I have suggested, to the relative contraindication of an interpretative approach. Furthermore, Blos (1962) has described the psychological task of late adolescence as one of character consolidation at which time the infantile conflicts are rendered specific and become centered within the self-representation. At this point, more traditional analytic work can proceed.

Geleerd (1957) has also noted that a consistent analysis of defense mechanisms is not desirable, and often contraindicated, in adolescence. Among other differences between adolescent and adult analysis, she also commented that the working-through process is limited, that transference is handled in a way to allow for a real relationship, and that there is a greater role in helping with reality-testing with the analyst acting at times as a parent substitute. All of these recommendations imply an approach that is not principally interpretative and that attempts to pace the relational shifts and integrative capacities in a particular adolescent. Anna Freud is quoted as saying, "One cannot analyze in adolescence. It is like running next to an express train" (Geleerd, 1957, p. 266). If analysis during the early phases of adolescence were formulated according to the specifies of the developmental phase, it might be seen that, in the "run next to the express train," analytic work was being accomplished in terms of a renegotiation of the paranoid-schizoid position. Thus when Geleerd states, "With this age group the emphasis is predominantly on the problems of daily life .... There appears to be a general poverty of material . . . and little communication of fantasy life"

(1957, p. 264). She is addressing, I believe, a relationship organized along schizoid themes. The aim of the therapeutic relationship is not to facilitate a special intimacy, but rather to facilitate a relationship in which distance is accepted. Support of defenses does not lie in well-articulated statements of support but in the context and structure of a relationship that can accommodate the developmentally limited capacity for relationship.

It has been suggested (Harley, 1970) that the limitations of psychoanalytic technique for the adolescent probably reflect a limitation of knowledge about the nature of adolescent psychopathology. A study of the more extreme manifestations of developmental psychopathology may serve to illuminate the processes of normal development. In the two cases which I briefly presented, the psychopathology was extreme, and the required psychotherapeutic technique was an exaggeration of what may be required for the less deviant adolescent. In formulating the early adolescent regression in terms of the Kleinian concept of the paranoid-schizoid position, I have emphasized the structure of experience and the capacity for relatedness which have direct bearing on the specific relationship in which psychotherapy will be elaborated. I believe that this consideration takes precedence over the specific conflictual themes associated with the various phases of adolescence (Blos, 1962b), the usefulness of which assumes a more-or-less insistently interpretative analytic approach. Content cannot be divorced from structure and the capacity for relatedness.

The less deviant adolescent will not show as fixed a regression as did the two adolescents I presented. His experience will shift between the earlier organization of the paranoid-schizoid position and the progressive depressive position of greater self and object stability. A radically different analytic approach is required in each of these early relational positions. The analyst who is aware of such differences will proceed with a greater clarity of therapeutic akin.

References

Blos, P. (1962a), *On Adolescence: A Psychoanalytic Interpretation*, Free Press, New York.

Blos, P. (1962b), Intensive psychotherapy in relation to the various phases of adolescence, in A. Esman (Ed.), *The Psychiatric Treatment of Adolescents*. International Universities Press, New York, 1983.

Blos, P. (1963), The concept of acting out in relation to the adolescent process, *J. Am. Acad. Child Psych.*, 2,118-136.

Coolidge, 1. C., Hahn, P. B., and Peck, A. L. (1957), School phobia: Neurotic crisis or way of life, *Am. J. Orthopsychiat.*, 27, 296-306.

Eisenberg, L. (1958), School phobia: a study in the communication of anxiety, *Am. J. Psychiat.*, 114, 712-718.

Erikson, E. H. (1968), *Identity Youth and Crisis*, Norton and Co., New York.

Fairbairn, W. R. D. (1940), Schizoid factors in the personality, in *Psychoanalytic Studies of the Personality*, Tavistock Publications, London, 1952.

Freud, A. (1958), Adolescence, *Psychoanal. Study Child.*, 13, 255-278.

Freud, S. (1905), Three essays on sexuality, in *Standard Edition*, Hogarth Press, London, 1955, Vol. 7, pp. 207-230.

Geleerd, E. (1957), Some aspects of psychoanalytic technique in adolescence, *Psychoanal.Study Child*, 12, 263-283.

Geleerd, E. (1961), Some aspects of ego vicissitudes in adolescence, *J. Am. Psychoanal. Assoc.*, 9, 394-405.

Group for the Advancement of Psychiatry (1968), *Normal Adolescence*, Scribners, New York.

Harley, M. (1961), Some observations on the relationship between genitality and structural development at adolescence, *J. Am. Psychoanal. Assoc.*, 9, 434-460.

Harley, M. (1970), On some problems of technique in the analysis of early adolescents, *Psychoanal. Study Child*, 25, 99-121.

Jacobson, E. (1964), *The Self and the Object World*, International Universities Press, New York.

Johnson, A., Falstein, E. I., and Szurek, S. A. (1941), School phobia, *Am. J. Orthopsychiatr.*, 11, 702-711.

Katan, A. (1951), The role of "displacement" in agoraphobia, *Int. J. Psychoanal*, 32, 41 -50.

Klein, G. (1976), *Psychoanalytic Theory*, International Universities Press,

New York.

Klein, M. (1932), The technique of analysis in puberty, in *The Psychoanalysis of Children*, Free Press, New York, 1984.

Klein, M. (1935), A contribution to the psychogenesis of manic-depressive states, in *Love, Guilt, and Reparation*, Free Press, New York, 1984.

Klein, M. (1946), Notes on some schizoid mechanisms, in *Envy and Gratitude*, Free Press, New York, 1984.

Laufer, M., and Laufer, M. E. (1984), *Adolescence and Developmental Breakdown*, Yale University Press, New Haven.

Ogden, T. (1986), *The Matrix of the Mind*, Jason Aronson, Northvale, N.J.

Segal, H. (1954), A note on schizoid mechanisms underlying phobia formation, *Int. J. Psychoanal.*, 35, 238-241.

Segal, H. (1981), *Melanie Klein*, Penguin Books, New York.

Sperling, M. (1967), School phobias, *Psychoanal. Study Child*, 22, 375-401.

CHAPTER SIXTEEN
A DEVELOPMENTAL
APPROACH TO THE
PSYCHOTHERAPY OF
ADOLESCENTS

Aaron Esman

As is well known, the first report of the psychoanalytic treatment of an adolescent was Freud's "Dora" case (1905). Freud's difficulty with the transference and countertransference issues in that case proved to be characteristic of the experience of many who have followed after him. His efforts to apply the psychoanalytic method to the treatment of adolescents were extended and applied in a more systematic, if highly modified, fashion by. August Aichhorn (1935), who established a residential treatment program for "wayward youth" based on Freud's principles. Aichhorn served as teacher and model to a generation of psychoanalytically trained educators such as Anna Freud, Erik Erikson, Peter Blos, Fritz Redl, Rudolf Ekstein, and others, who brought with them the principles of analytically oriented psychotherapy with adolescents when they left Vienna. More recently, workers such as Bruch (1979), Laufer (1977), Masterson (1972), and others have expanded the range of adolescent psychotherapy to the borderline disorders, eating disorders, and "developmental breakdowns" that may characterize this phase. In addition, group (Berkovitz,1972), family (Williams, 1973), and behavioral (Lehrer, Schiff, and Kris, 1971) methods have been developed for special application to adolescent patients. I shall not consider these valuable methods here, for both lack of time and lack of expertise. I shall focus, rather, on ambulatory, individual, psychodynamically oriented psychotherapy-the kind of work which, I suspect, for most of us makes up the bulk of our professional activity with our youthful patients.

Psychotherapy with Adolescents

Adolescence is, by definition, a transitional period. Its onset can, for most purposes, be arbitrarily defined as concurrent with puberty, but its end point is vague and indeterminate, shading off as it does into whatever a particular culture defines, by various criteria, as adulthood (Blos 1977). Rapid and kaleidoscopic change characterizes the period, manifest in every sphere of life-physical, cognitive, affective, and social. Accordingly the techniques of psychotherapy must also vary as the adolescent progresses in the subphases of this protean and mercurial stage of growth. A developmental approach to the subject is, therefore, in order-one which correlates the therapeutic principles and the developmental needs and tasks of the growing person.

Blos (1962) has outlined some of the issues that apply here, emphasizing the intrapsychic factors that accompany these developmental shifts. This discussion will, in some respects, be an elaboration of his seminal contribution, but I shall, perhaps, paint with a broader brush. I shall attempt to delineate, not so much pathological variants, but the normally occurring expectable features of adolescent development that must affect our technical approaches to our patients.

INDICATIONS

A few words about the indications for the kind of treatment I am concerned with here. The adolescent who can, in principle at least, make use of ambulatory, psychoanalytically oriented psychotherapy is the nonpsychotic youngster whose symptoms and/or behavioral difficulties are not so severe as to preclude continuation of life in the community the mildly, to moderately depressed youngster who is actively experimenting with drugs but is not an addict; the academic underachiever who may or may not have a true learning disability but whose capacity to concentrate on his work is interfered with by anxiety or preoccupying thoughts; the anxious, socially inhibited adolescent; the adolescent whose behavioral difficulties-petty thievery, sexual promiscuity-seem on assessment to be derivatives of chronic, phase-related, intrapsychic conflict rather than manifestations of a sociopathic character disorder, the adolescent who is having difficulty in adapting to change in parental circumstances such as death or separation, divorce or remarriage. In addition many adolescents whose rebelliousness, eating disorders, or overanxious behavior reveals them to be caught in the web of inextricably interwoven family conflicts may require and benefit from such individual therapy in addition to concurrent treatment focused on the family system itself.

EARLY ADOLESCENCE

I shall begin our developmental survey with a description of the subphase characteristics of the early adolescent, that is, the young person between the ages of about twelve and about fourteen. Persons in this age group are, at least in my experience, exceptionally difficult to engage in any individual exploratory psychotherapy. Some of the reasons for this difficulty are as follows:

1. The early adolescent is operat under intense drive pressure stimulated both by the pubertal activation of his endocrine system and, by the sociocultural pressures attendant on the prevailing stereotypes of adolescent behavior as transmitted through the "media." This pressure is experienced with relation not only to sexual but to aggressive impulses and their derivatives as well. It is manifested behaviorally in a powerful action orientation; the early adolescent is not ordinarily disposed to deal with his internal tensions and conflicts by reflection or introspection but rather by action on and in his environment. Since psychoanalytic psychotherapy asks of its subjects the suspension of motor activity and the direction of attention toward internal mental processes, its demands are out of phase with the customary direction of early adolescent physical and psychological pressures.

2. A primary issue for the early adolescent is the protector of his nascent and still very tenuous sense of autonomy as he begins to break out of the relatively compliant position of normal latency and to test out his newfound strengths and competencies. The early adolescent rarely comes to treatment on his own initiative; he is usually brought by parents or sent by some authoritative institution such as the school or the court. In either case, he is likely to be mistrustful of those adults whom he sees as attempting to impinge upon or restrict his shaky sense of self-determination. In most circumstances he is likely to see the therapist as yet another such adult, an agent of his parents and/or the community institution that is attempting to impose itself upon him. He is likely, therefore, to relate initially to the therapist with suspicion and mistrust.

3. Offer (1969) and his associates, among others, have by now exploded the myth of "normal" adolescent turmoil. We know now that despite the well-known stresses of this phase, the modal adolescent succeeds in passing through this developmental transition without major psychological disruption. It is still true, however, that in early adolescence some turmoil and rebelliousness normally occur if only with respect to minor issues bearing on personal autonomy such as length of hair, curfew hours, and so

forth. Along with this transitory rebelliousness the early adolescent, in part because of his preoccupation with the changes that are occurring in his body and their psychic elaboration, is primarily self-oriented. Those persons relied on for interaction and emotional support are likely to be his peers rather than adults-that is, people whom he sees as like himself, sharing his concerns, and testing out the same issues. None of these-his rebelliousness, his narcissism, or his peer orientation-is likely to dispose him toward a relationship with a strange, intrusive adult.

4. One of the principal concerns-indeed, in the view of some, the principal concern-of the early adolescent is the mastery of his rising sexual fantasies and his conflicts around the pressure to masturbate. These are the natural and inevitable reactions to puberty and the awakening of genital sensations. In Laufer's (1977) view, it is precisely the ability to accept with comfort the "sexual body" and to permit guilt-free masturbation with full integration of pregenital and genital fantasy that is the essence of successful adolescent development. For most young adolescents, however, these impulses and fantasies are the source of intense feelings of shame and/or guilt despite the dissemination of factual information about the normality and inevitability of such feelings and wishes. It is difficult in the extreme for young adolescents to discuss these matters with anybody, even their peers. It is particularly difficult for them to discuss them with a strange adult, especially one of the opposite sex who may be seen as a surrogate for the parents who are the subject, consciously or unconsciously, of their forbidden fantasies.

5. The defensive structure of the early adolescent tends to be quite rigid, maintaining to a considerable degree the characteristic late latency reliance on denial and externalization as major defensive measures. This defensive rigidity is related, I believe, to the dominant cognitive mode characterizing most people in this age group. Although Piaget (1969) has placed the onset of formal operational thought in the twelve to fifteen age period, it is clear, as demonstrated by Dulit (1972), that many, if not most adolescents, even unusually intelligent and highly educated groups, do not achieve this cognitive pattern at least until mid adolescence, if at all. Accordingly. the usual early adolescent remains somewhat concrete in his thinking and tends to be present oriented rather than capable of reflecting on his past and anticipating his future. Since psychoanalytic psychotherapy expects of its participants the ability to do both of these things, the capacity of those who remain fixed in the stage of concrete operational thought to engage in such therapy is limited.

These normal developmental aspects of early adolescence have significant implications for the technique of psychotherapy. Above all, they dictate a high degree of flexibility regarding procedural and technical arrangements with the pubertal and just postpubertal patient. These young people generally require of the therapist a degree of activity higher than that which is customary for older patients. Above all, they have an intense intolerance for silences, since these tend to throw them back on their own affectively charged fantasies and to leave them with the sense of being unsupported. It is incumbent on the therapist to be more present, or, if you will, "realer" than he is likely to be with his adult patients or, indeed, even with latency-age children. At times, the early adolescent who is uncomfortable with the relative passivity of the psychotherapeutic situation or is so guarded as to be unable to participate in verbal exchange may need to resort to child therapy techniques, such as game playing or model making in order to preserve therapeutic contact.

A cautionary note should be introduced here, however. Many therapists of adolescents operate with the belief that, like some of those portrayed in films, they should relate to their adolescent patients as "pals," affecting casual dress, using adolescent lingo-, and ostentatiously demonstrating their familiarity and comfort with adolescent folkways. In my view, this is a serious error and one likely to lead to unforeseen and unfortunate consequences. In the long run, the adolescent patient does not want his therapist to be a peer but a sympathetic and understanding adult. No one is more sensitive to in authenticity than a young adolescent, and he is almost certain to identify such behavior on the therapist's part as spurious and seductive. I cannot, therefore, urge too strongly the maintenance by the therapist of his adult identity and the integrity of his professional status.

The establishment of the therapeutic alliance with the young adolescent is likely to take a lone time. Most such patients are slow to trust an will require what Blos has referred to as a "preparatory phase" of uncertain duration before they can begin to understand the nature of psychotherapy and enter into a true therapeutic process. During this preparatory phase, the therapist must be prepared to meet his patient at the latter's own level.

This is likely to mean spending many hours listening to what the therapist may be inclined to regard as superficial chitchat about phase-typical preoccupations. Girls are likely to talk endlessly about the vicissitudes of their peer relationships and their newfound interest in clothes and makeup. Boys are likely to spend many hours talking about sports and the latest horror movies. The therapist who cannot under these conditions maintain an interest in his patient and a genuine awareness of the importance of these issues in the everyday life of the young adolescent is likely to have a difficult time engendering in him a sense of real empathy and shared concern.

The early adolescent is likely to be a very busy person. He is, as I noted earlier, primarily oriented toward action in a wide variety of spheres In addition, particularly if he is of middle- or upper-class origin, his parents will have ambitions and concerns for him that transcend the therapeutic situation. Accordingly, he is likely to be involved with a wide range of activities that will make extensive demands on his time. Activities such as soccer games, track meets, piano lessons, appointments with the orthodontist, rehearsals for the school play, choral performances, preparation for Bar Mitzvah-all these will be of the most urgent importance in the young adolescent's life and will encroach on the time available for psychotherapy appointments. Together with the early adolescent's guardedness and reserve about the whole therapeutic procedure and his need to preserve his sense of autonomy and self-determination these activities are likely to lead to frequent cancellations, demands for alternative appointments, and failures to appear at scheduled times. The therapist of the early adolescent must be prepared and must prepare the family for such eventualities. If he wishes to maintain his relationship with his patient he must, again, be prepared to be flexible about his time arrangements, be willing to change appointments and schedule makeups and tolerate with reasonably good humor the inevitable cancellations and no-shows. On the other hand, it must be clear both to the patient and to the family that the therapist is entitled to compensation for his time and that the patient and the family must be responsible for scheduled sessions In other words, the therapist must be flexible but not infinitely manipulable or masochistic with respect to the complicated and shifting scheduling requirements of his adolescent patient.

Above all, the therapist of the young adolescent is well advised to maintain a developmental orientation toward his therapeutic goals. Even when impelled by subjective distress, the young adolescent is likely, to be interested in the therapeutic process only to the extent it addresses itself to those particular problems interfering with his normal developmental progression. Once his symptoms or maladaptive behavioral difficulties resolved in the course of therapy, it is unlikely that he will have further interest in continuing therapeutic contact. Remember, he is likely, if he is a patient amenable to this therapeutic approach at all, to be a busy person with many competing interests. The therapist should, therefore, be prepared to accept limited objectives and to regard symptom relief as a legitimate therapeutic goal. Strategically, he should be agreeable to the notion of brief or interrupted episodes of therapy rather than striving for unrealizable goals of major personality transformation. A corollary of this is the likelihood that, except for the more passive patient, few early adolescents will be amenable to the extended and regression-inducing procedure of classical psychoanalytic therapy.

Finally, a note about the role of the therapist's sex. There are few circumstances in which I would regard the sex of the therapist to be a critical issue in the therapeutic process. In most situations, both maternal and paternal elements of transference paradigms can be experienced and worked with irrespective of the therapist's actual sex. The one exception to this view is that of the early adolescent patient. As indicated above, the critical phase-specific preoccupation of early adolescents with their nascent sexuality and their masturbatory conflicts is invested with feelings of shame and the potential for humiliation that make it difficult in the extreme for them to communicate with an adult of the opposite sex. Further, the proximity to consciousness of oedipal wishes and fantasies makes the opposite-sex therapist a potentially dangerous figure for many early adolescent patients. For these reasons I believe that, wherever possible, young adolescents are best treated by a therapist of the same sex. Where this is not feasible, of course, therapy should not wait on the unavailable therapist, but the process is more likely to proceed productively when such arrangements can be worked out.

MID ADOLESCENCE

So much for the problem of the young adolescent. What about the young person in the next subphase-that of mid adolescence, or, as Blos refers to it, "adolescence proper"-the period between about fifteen to about eighteen, that is, the high school years? Here again, subphase-specific characteristics will tend to shape ways in which the therapeutic interaction proceeds and the technical approach that the therapist brings to his work.

The healthy mid adolescent is likely to have arrived at some reasonable accommodation to his pubertal development. He is more comfortable with his body and more accustomed to the sensations and fantasies that his pubescence has generated. As a result, he is likely to be less rigidly narcissistic and better able to interact empathically with others than is his younger sibling. Although he is still relatively action oriented. he is under considerably less impulse pressure and is better able to engage in introspection and delay of gratification than he was at twelve or thirteen. Further, given the fact of his increased physical maturation and the likelihood under normal circumstances of his having been granted more opportunities for independent action, he is likely to be more secure about his developing autonomy and, therefore, less guarded and suspicious of the motives of adults. This being the case, he is less likely to employ rigid and relatively primitive defenses and, on the other hand, more likely to recognize and acknowledge subjective distress than the younger adolescent. Although he is still deeply engaged in his peer culture, he is, as Ianni (1983) has recently demonstrated, more likely than he had been earlier to turn to adults for support and guidance in areas of value formation and the planning of his future. Indeed, it is during this period, as his cognitive development proceeds in the direction of formal operational thought and as his perception of reality becomes better consolidated, that he begins to think seriously about his future and about the potential consequences of his current behaviors. Serious consideration of vocational goals becomes a feature of this period and, along with the mid-adolescent preoccupation with values, ideals, and abstract philosophical concerns may engender a need for the active support and guidance of valued and trusted adults.

Despite all these progressive developmental characteristics, however it should be recognized that the normal mid adolescent may be prey to shifting moods and to a dysphoric diathesis as he steers his course through the gradual process of "object removal"-that is, the revision of his earlier intense attachment to his parents and the ultimate establishment of mature connections with nonincestuous love objects. Many will be exquisitely sensitive to rejections or losses that leave them feeling objectless and alone; under these circumstances, even the relatively healthy adolescent may experience depressive moments and entertain transient suicidal thoughts. Further, the normal mid adolescent is still capable of regressive movements that Blos believes are a necessary aspect of adolescent development. It is certainly true that premature consolidation of advanced developmental positions without the flexibility that allows for change, experimentation, and revision of identifications constitutes a significant restriction of the optimal unfolding of the personality. Still, one should be aware that even the most mature-appearing mid adolescent is capable of regressing from thoughtful introspection to frenetic activity, particularly where resistance can be rationalized as being adaptively appropriate. I recall, for instance, the case of an extraordinarily bright and gifted fifteen-year-old girl, the product of an enormously complex family of mixed racial origin and radical political orientation, who came to treatment in the throes of a moderately severe depression that was significantly interfering with her academic and social life. Consistent with her family background, she was deeply interested in the antinuclear movement and spent a considerable amount of time in treatment talking about her involvement with various aspects of the then current campaign against the development of nuclear reactors. She proceeded quite well in therapy, however, and was deeply engaged in examining her feelings about her relations with her parents and her profound sense of disappointment and disillusionment in them. When the Three Mile Island incident occurred, this girl was galvanized into activity. She became energized by the activation of the movement around this near disaster and profoundly immersed in a series of demonstrations, marches, and protests that came in its wake. Her depression lifted, and it became clear that she had no time in her busy schedule for the luxury of psychotherapy. She thanked me for my help and made it clear that life was now offering her more in terms of purpose and fulfillment than I was able to give her. That, in sum, was the end of her psychotherapy.

All of these developmental trends have influence on the principles of technique in our work with mid-adolescent patients. We are no longer likely to require the use of nonverbal child therapy devices to promote communication, although there may be special cases of withdrawn schizoid adolescents who may require and benefit from the use of such games as chess, as described forty years ago by Fleming and Strong (1943) as a means of establishing contact while maintaining a protective distance. Normally, the communicative process in the treatment of the mid adolescent will be essentially a conversational one, though still one that will require from the therapist more activity than he may be accustomed to employing with his adult patients. As indicated earlier, the mid-adolescent is likely to be in quest of guidance and clarification around issues of values, morality, and ideals. The therapist may, therefore, have to express himself directly on such matters without attempting to impose his views on his patient. This may come up particularly around such matters as drug taking, sexual behavior, and the like. A due respect for the adolescent's autonomy and his phase appropriate efforts to forge his own sense of identity will dictate both the therapeutic focus and the therapist's tactful, though frank, response.

Nonetheless, there may be occasions in the treatment of all adolescents- but particularly the mid adolescent- when active, limit-setting intervention on the therapist's part is not only advisable but essential. The mid adolescent's normative depressive propensity may, in a disturbed adolescent, advance to the point of active suicidal ideation or behavior; his normal experimental tendency may carry him so far as to involve him in behaviors that threaten his health or even his survival. In such instances the therapist must be prepared to act decisively and appropriately to protect his patient from the consequences of the miscarried extremity of his phase-related dispositions and his still imperfectly developed impulse control.

The mid-adolescent probably poses the greatest challenge of any patient to the therapist's ability to monitor and regulate his countertransference responses. Anthony (1969) has written convincingly about the reactions of adults to adolescents and their tendency to stereotype adolescent behavior in response to the anxieties that it arouses in them. In this respect the therapist is not likely to be different from other adults. He must constantly be on guard against the danger of being seduced into recapitulating with the adolescent behaviors to which the latter is accustomed in his transactions with people in his everyday life. This applies to both sexual and aggressive responses. Two polar positions may be assumed by an unwary therapist in reaction to such seductions, either of which can have disastrous consequences. The first is that of over identification with the adolescent and concomitant hostility toward parents and other authoritative figures whom the patient and then the therapist see as oppressing him. This would be equivalent to the parental stance that "I was like that when I was a kid and I turned out all right." The second is overidentification with parents and authority figures and concomitant hostility to the adolescent himself. This would be the corollary of the parental position that "I couldn't get away with that stuff when I was his age and I don't see any reason why he should either." In either case, the therapist is likely to be responding not so much to the realities of the patient's situation and behavior but to unresolved adolescent conflicts of his own that the patient's behavior reactivates. Constant self-scrutiny, therefore, is a necessary condition for psychotherapeutic work with adolescents at all stages-but particularly during this crucial mid-adolescent period.

LATE ADOLESCENCE

About the older adolescent, the eighteen- to twenty-one-year-old college age youth, there is less specifically to be said. He is fully matured physically, frequently well advanced into higher-level cognitive functioning, and at least potentially capable of self-observation and introspection. The college-age adolescent who is otherwise suitable or psychoanalytically oriented psychotherapy can be treated, from a technical standpoint very much in the manner of an adult. At this age, classical psychoanalytic technique can more frequently be employed, and the therapist may assume a less active, more observant stance than he is likely to be able to use with the younger adolescent. Special circumstances will arise here again, related to phase-appropriate developmental needs where considerations of going away to college or graduate education conflict with continuing in or initiating therapy in a particular geographic locale. In such instances, therapeutic needs must be carefully balanced against appropriate developmental advances, but the ultimate decision should, except in emergency situations, be left after appropriate reflection to the maturing adolescent himself. In most cases, alternative therapeutic arrangements can be made even in what seem relatively remote settings. One does not wish to present the adolescent with a situation in which he must view leaving as an act of rebellion or staying as an act of submission (although, of course, in the transference he may well do so).

I want to emphasize again what you all know-that all adolescents are likely to be provocative and constantly to test the therapist's commitment and his neutrality. The therapist must respond with, in Trilling's (1972) terms, "sincerity and authenticity" if he is to engender credibility with adolescent patients. The therapist must be prepared for the fact that only in rare instances can he anticipate anything resembling a full resolution of the transference in his therapeutic work with adolescents. Indeed, recent studies by Firestein (1978), Pfeffer (1974), and others seriously question the possibility of such full transference resolution in even the most intensive analytic work with adults. But certainly in work with adolescents, one has to be prepared to do "pieces" of therapy addressed to specific and limited conflictual areas, making knowing use of positive transference configurations and recognizing that, in many instances, the exploration of negative transference issues and the ultimate resolution of those negative oedipal residues that Blos (1977) regards as crucial for the attainment of true adult status must await more intensive and systematic exploration at a later time. Certain fundamental therapeutic dicta apply particularly to work with all adolescents, particularly that dictum which prescribes interpretive work directed primarily at maladaptive defenses rather than, or at least considerably prior to, attempts at unearthing pathogenic instinctual conflicts.

THE ROLE OF THE FAMILY

Finally, a few words about the role of parents. I believe that in any work with an adolescent, at least one who is either physically or financially dependent on parents, the latter should be seen initially with, of course, the permission of the patient, and with or without his or her presence, as he or she chooses. Not only is valuable information to be obtained from such meetings, but I believe that parents have the right to see the person to whom they are entrusting the care of their child and to whom they are paying what is usually a substantial fee. On the other hand, for mid and late adolescents, I prefer to see the patient first, whenever possible, in order to emphasize my position that I am there to take care of him rather than to deal with his parents' complaints. Similarly, I discourage parents from making appointment arrangements for their adolescents; I prefer to make such arrangements directly with the patient as a way of recognizing the real demands that they have on their schedules and their growing self-regulation. Although family therapy is frequently useful as a mode of treatment for adolescents, in the kind of treatment I am discussing parents are not regularly or systematically included in the treatment process. I do, however, find that it is useful in specific circumstances to arrange family meetings where clarification of obscure issues and resolution of specific situational conflicts are frequently possible. I am very protective, however, of the confidentiality of my patients' communications and make it clear from the outset that whatever they tell me remains with us, whereas whatever their parents tell me is not so protected. I feel free to communicate to the adolescent anything that his parents have told me so as to make it clear that no collusion exists between them and me and that he has a right to know whatever concerns him. Finally, and as a matter of course, it appears to me that where parents need sustained work either as a couple or individually, or where family therapy is indicated, I should make no effort to conduct such treatment myself but refer them to others. I believe that my ability to focus my attention on the adolescent himself, and his ability to see me as his working collaborator, would be compromised were I to attempt to be everyone's therapist at once.

In considering these comments about family involvement, I have come to realize that I am speaking from a special and perhaps unusual perspective-the perspective of one who practices in the center of a great metropolis richly endowed with public transit facilities that make it possible for even early adolescents to make and keep appointments on their own. For those in other, less favored communities where the adolescent, at least until driving age, is dependent on parents for transportation to and from his sessions, the situation will be quite different and, I believe, less desirable. There one does not enjoy the prerogative of choice as to whether the patient comes alone to his initial session; one may not even be able to schedule such an appointment-or any appointment at all- without considering the complexities of parental schedules, and, if both parents work, these may be complicated indeed. And, as one colleague put it, "as often as not it is the parents who cancel the kid's appointment because they're sick or have something else to do." Having largely been spared these problems, I can say little about their management except to underscore both the inevitable need for flexibility and the inherent limitations that such circumstances impose on the therapeutic process in work with younger adolescents. Certainly the goal that many of us set-the promotion of the adolescent's functioning and his sense of a truly autonomous self-is not favored by such practical reinforcements of his dependent status.

Conclusions

Let me, in concluding, then, state what I regard as the essential elements of the climate of the therapeutic encounter in work with adolescents. I believe that the therapist's stance should be one of openness without inauthentic self-exposure, of empathy without overidentification or loss of appropriate distance, of respect for the patient's autonomy without affective detachment, and, finally, of flexibility without abandoning fundamental therapeutic principles. A lightness of touch need not conflict with, but should not subvert, a seriousness of purpose-that purpose being the restoration to the adolescent of his normal, phase-appropriate development and function. In a climate such as this, I believe the adolescent can grow, can resolve crippling inhibitions and revise maladaptive defenses, and can, where his basic psychic organization permits, return to a healthy developmental track. Psychotherapy cannot insure against later difficulties, nor can it undo the corrosive effects of social disorganization and deprivation. As physicians and psychiatrists, however, we have the means to alleviate needless suffering for many troubled adolescents and their families if we but use it wisely and well.

REFERENCES

Aichhorn, A. 1935. *Wayward Youth*. New York: Viking, 1948.
Anthony, E. J. 1969. The reactions of adults to adolescents and their behavior. In A. H. Esman, ed. *The Psychology of Adolescence*. New York:

International Universities Press, 1975.

Berkovitz, I. 1972. *Adolescents Grow in Groups*. New York: Brunner/ Mazel.

Blos, P. 1962. Intensive psychotherapy in relation to the various phases of the adolescent period. *American Journal of Orthopsychiatry* 32:901-910.

Blos, P. 1976. When and how does adolescence end? *Adolescent Psychiatry* 5:5-17.

Bruch, H. 1979. Island in the river: the anorexic adolescent in treatment. Adolescent Psychiatry 7:26-40.

Dulit, E. 1972. Adolescent thinking a la Piaget: the formal stage. *Journal of Youth and Adolescence* 1:281-301

Firestein, S. 1978. *Termination in Psychoanalysis*. New York: International Universities Press.

Fleming, J., and Strong, D. 1943. Observation on the use of chess in the treatment of an adolescent boy. *Psychoanalytic Review* 30:399-416.

Freud, S. 1905. Fragment of the analysis of a case of hysteria. *Standard Edition* 7:7-122. London: Hogarth, 1953.

Ianni, F. 1983. *Home, School and Community in Adolescent Education*. Washington: U.S. Department of Education.

Laufer, M. 1975. Preventive intervention in adolescence. *Psychoanalytic Study of the Child* 30:511-528.

Laufer, M. 1977 A view of adolescent pathology. *Adolescent Psychiatry* 5:243-256.

Lehrer, P.; Schiff, L.; and Kris, A. 1971. Operant conditioning in a comprehensive treatment program for adolescents. *Archives of General Psychiatry* 25:515-521.

Masterson, J. 1972. Treatment of the Borderline Adolescent: A Developmental Approach. New York. Wiley.

Offer, D. 1969. The Psychological World of the Teenager: A Study of Normal Adolescent Development. New York:Basic.

Piaget, J. 1969. The intellectual development of the adolescent. In A. H. Esman, ed.The Psychology of Adolescence. New York: International universities Press, 1975.

Pfeffer, A. 1974. The fate of the transference neurosis after analysis. *Journal of the American Psychoanalytic Association* 22: 895- 903.

Trilling, L. 1972. *Sincerity and Authenticity*. Cambridge, Mass.: Harvard University Press.

Williams, F. 1973. Family therapy: its role in adolescent psychiatry. *Adolescent Psychiatry* 2:324-329.

INDEX

Wertham, S., 142
White, R., 136
White Institute, 82, 213
Wieder, H., 152
Williams, F., 247
Wineman, D., 11
Winnicott, D., 3, 14, 15, 16, 17,
21, 148
Withdrawal, 44, 45, 235, 236
Withdrawing part unit, 195-197
Wittels, F., 51
Wynne, L., 102
Zetzel, E., 57, 68
Zinner, J., 16

ABOUT THE EDITOR

James B. McCarthy, Ph.D. is a psychologist and psychoanalyst in private practice in Forest Hills and Manhattan, New York. He is Director of Psychology and Coordinator of Professional Training, Queens Children's Psychiatric Center, a faculty member and supervisor at the Manhattan Institute for Psychoanalysis and St. John's University and has been on the faculty of New York University, Yeshiva University and New York Medical College. He is the author of *Death Anxiety: The Loss of the Self* (1980), *Adolescence and Character Disturbance* (1994) and many papers on borderline and psychotic patients and child and adolescent psychotherapy.